The Yoga
of Mind
Control

Mind Power Secrets
of the Ancient Yogis

Yogacharya Michael Deslippe

2nd Edition

Edited By: Edit This One, LLC, P.O. Box 172, Fairfax, IA 52228 www.editTHISone.com

Published in the United States by: Edit This One, LLC d/b/a Wordy Gerty Publishing

The publisher does not have any control over and does not assume any responsibility for author or third-party websites or their content.

Published using: CreateSpace Paperback and KDP Publishing, both are Amazon.com companies.

Printed By: Eagle Book Bindery, Cedar Rapids, IA

ISBN: 978-0-9981046-1-4

Dedication

This publication is dedicated to the great Dr. Swami Gitananda Giri Gurumaharaj of Pondicherry India, whose teachings have inspired and enlightened so many along the path of Yoga.

Table of Contents

It gives me great pleasure to write a few words of appreciation and admiration for one of my dearest yoga friends, a brother in yoga who has such a deep understanding of this great art and science. Yogacharya Michael has understood the true nature of Yoga and is making a great effort to propagate it in its pristine purity through the modern facility of the Internet. This is a true union of the ancient and the new for the teachings are as ancient as they can be, yet, the methods of instruction are the most modern possible.

May my Guru and father, Yogamaharishi Dr. Swami Gitananda Giri Guru Maharaj and my beloved Guru and mother, Ammaji, Meenakshi Devi Bhavanani bless us all for the success of this noble endeavor to spread the message of classical yoga to all nooks and corners of the world.

As this book deals with the concept of the mind, and yoga has a lot to say on this topic, I feel it would be apt for me to pen a few words on the basic concepts of yoga psychology that are the foundation for conscious living.

The art and science of Yoga may be defined as a process, or journey, as well as a state of being, or the goal of the journey. It is first and foremost the science and art of quieting our subconscious mind – though it is also a way of life, skill in action, union of thought, word and deed and an integration of our personality at all levels. It is the science of conscious evolution and is also the process of attaining the ultimate state of emotional and mental equanimity itself.

Yoga is one of the greatest treasures of our unique Indian cultural heritage and it enables us to develop a clear understanding of the human mind. Yoga treats the human being as a multi-layered, conscious being, possessing three bodies *(sthula, sukshma and kaarana sharira)* and being enveloped in a five-layered *(pancha kosha)* existence. This ancient science of mind control as codified by Maharishi Patanjali more than 2500 years ago helps us to understand our mental processes as well as the cause – effect relations of a multitude of problems facing modern humankind.

The mind is considered to have four internal processes or *antahkarana*. These processes are the memory bank or the subconscious data storage center *(chitta)*, the conscious mind dealing with everyday stuff *(manas)*, the discerning intellect *(buddhi)* and the ego principle *(ahamkara)* (consisting of the impure ego that feels all is ME and MINE as well as the pure ego which understands that all is MINE as a manifestation of the Divine). The *buddhi* is further said to possess three powers: the power of will *(iccha Shakti)*, the power of action *(kriya Shakti)*, and the power of wisdom *(jnana Shakti)*. In the yogic scheme of things, it is most important that all these powers work together in synchrony for otherwise there will be disaster. The *chitta bhumi* or states of the mind consist of the undeveloped, inert mind that is as dull as stone *(mudha)*, the totally distracted state of mind *(kshipta)*, the partially distracted state of mind *(vikshipta)*, the concentrated state of mind *(ekagratha)* and the controlled mind of the true yogi *(niruddha)*.

The worldly person always feels that their problem lies elsewhere and that they are the innocent victim of circumstances and fate. Yoga teaches us that most of our problems lie within us and that we have to undergo conscious change in order to solve them. Our

Guru, Yogamaharishi Dr. Swami Gitananda Giri used to often tell his students, *"You don't have any problem – YOU are the problem!"*

The modifications or fluctuations of the mind stuff are of five types, as described by Maharishi Patanjali in his classic yoga text, *The Yoga Sutras*. These are: cognition *(pramana)*, misconception *(viparyaya)*, imagination *(vikalpa)*, sleep *(nidra)*, and memory *(smrithi)*. He also states that when the mind is not controlled there is identification with these vrittis *(vritti sarupyam itarate)* and that the whole process of Yoga is aimed at *chittavritti nirodhah*, the "cessation of the whirlpools of the mind," in order that we are established in our true self *(swarupevastaanam)*. Patanjali elucidates the key to success as a dedicated and determined practice *(abhyasa)* coupled with a dispassionate and detached attitude towards everything *(vairagya)*.

Whereas, the worldly man fears hell and aspires for a heaven to be attained after death, the yogi realizes that heaven and hell are no more than planes of consciousness. Heaven and hell lie within us and it is for us to determine whether we want our life to be heaven or hell, for ourselves and for those around us.

While the worldly man searches for happiness in the pursuit of external experiences, the Yogi realizes that supreme happiness *(paramanandam)* lies within our inner being and that we only need to realize the folly of looking for happiness outside to be truly happy. True contentment *(santhosha)*, one of the five ethical observances of *Ashtanga Yoga (pancha niyama)* is the key to unexcelled happiness. Pujya Swamiji used to say, *"Health and Happiness are your birthright – claim them! Don't' barter them away for the plastics of the modern world."*

According to Maharishi Patanjali, most of our problems stem from the five psycho-physiological afflictions *(pancha klesha)* that are inborn in each and every human being. These five hindrances to spiritual growth are ignorance *(avidya),* egoism *(asmita)* and our sense of needing to survive at any cost *(abinivesha)* as well as the attraction *(raaga)* to external objects and the repulsion *(dwesha)* to them. Ignorance *(avidya)* is usually the start of most problems along with the ego *(asmita).* Then, our sense of needing to survive at any cost *(abinivesha)* compounds it further. Both attraction *(raaga)* to external objects and the repulsion *(dwesha)* to them need to be destroyed in order to attain tranquility as well as equanimity of emotions and the mind. Maharishi Patanjali further states that the practice of Yoga of mental purification *(Kriya Yoga)* consisting of disciplined effort *(tapas),* self analysis *(swadhyaya)* and surrender to the Divine will *(ishwara pranidhana)* is the means to destroy these five mental afflictions and attain to the state of *Samadhi* or oneness with the Supreme Self of the Divine.

The yogic concepts of mental and emotional equanimity *(samatvam)* and the even minded, balanced human being *(stitha prajna)* give us role models that we may strive to emulate. An understanding of the *pancha klesha* and their role in the creation of stress and the stress response help us to know our self better and understand the how's and why's of what we do. The concept of the *pancha kosha* – the five-layered existence of man as elucidated in the Taittiriya Upanishad – helps us to understand that we have more than only the physical existence and also gives us an insight into the role of the mind in causation of our physical problems and psychosomatic disorders. All of these concepts help us to look at life with a different perspective – a view we call *yoga drishti* – and strive to evolve consciously toward becoming **human** beings.

Yoga helps us to take the right attitude toward our problems and thus tackle them in an effective manner. "To have the will *(iccha Shakti)* to change *(kriya Shakti)* that which can be changed, the strength to accept that which can not be changed, and the wisdom *(jnana Shakti)* to know the difference" is the attitude that needs to be cultivated. An attitude of letting go of worries and problems, and a greater understanding of our mental process helps to create a harmony in our body and mind whose disharmony is the main cause of *aadi-vyadhi,* or psychosomatic disorders.

The Yogis wish peace and happiness not only for themselves, but also for all beings on all the different planes of existence. They are not individualists seeking salvation for only themselves, but on the contrary are **universalists** seeking to live life in the proper evolutionary manner to the best of their ability and with care and concern for their human brethren as well as all beings on all planes of existence.

"Om, Loka Samasta Sukhino Bhavanthu Sarve
Janaha Sukhino Bhavanthu"

"Om Shanti, Shanti, Shanti, Om"

Yogacharya Dr. Ananda Balayogi Bhavanani
Chairman: Yoganjali Natyalayam and International Center for Yoga Education and Research (ICYER)
Hon General Secretary: Pondicherry Yogasana Association

RENE DESCARTES, the French scientist and philosopher said, "I think, therefore I am," a now famous remark that has become synonymous with the enigmatic relationship between mind and being. The ancient yogis have always understood this inter-relationship, though they may not exactly agree with his assertion. They may perhaps say something more like, "I am, therefore I think!" Either way, thought plays a fundamental role in this experience we call, "life."

It is widely accepted in modern psychology that how we think – our attitudes, outlook and mindset – has a definite effect on what we are able to achieve in life. The power of positive thinking is also at the foundation of pretty much all of the most popular new age self-help and personal improvement strategies, like: *The 7 Habits of Highly Effective People, How to Win Friends and Influence People,* and *The Secret,* just to name a few. In fact, at the heart of any strategy for productive change is one thing – changing the way you think.

But can the manner, quality and type of thoughts that we have go beyond just the results that we get out of life and also influence "what" or "who" we actually are? The yogis believed so, and they not only had a logical, scientific way of explaining why, but also a practical process for helping us to, as the US ARMY put it, "Be all you can be."

Our ancient yogic scientist, known as Rishis, also discovered that our thoughts could even extend beyond our own self to influence others and the environment around us. Many psychics, spiritualist and metaphysicians today also make these claims with ideas such as remote healing or the power to influence people and events through collective, mental efforts alone. But, is it true and does it really work? According to the ancient Rishis, it definitely does. More importantly; however, these powers are not only the domain of occultisms and the faithful, they rest with equal potential within all of us and the yogis discovered exactly how to unlock that potent force. This book is an unveiling of that knowledge.

The Mental Side of Yoga

Even thousands of years ago, Yoga Masters understood the effectiveness of thought, its power to propel one to the highest of spiritual achievements, or conversely, into utter annihilation. They interwove those realizations into the fabric of their ancient Indian culture so that even the average person who was not inclined to delve deeply into the spiritual life could still live a dignified and evolutionary life. The remnants of those realizations are still evident in the culture of modern day India, behaviors that, to the Western observer, may seem strange or be misinterpreted as irrational or even superstitious.

But global cultures today, even in India, have moved far away from their ancient foundations, structures that were built upon a higher sense of purpose and a deeper understanding of our hidden, universal nature. Today, especially in Western cultures, the notion that a powerful potential for personal and global transformation lies in gaining a deeper understanding of ourselves does not register with much importance. In fact, few today give even a meager moments pause to consider how something as ordinary as "thought" impacts their life or the lives of others – or even the state of the world around them.

The Yoga MIND CONTROL METHOD (working title only) will show you how it does. This book is not a flaky depiction of mystical magical techniques, or a jumbled expose of pseudo-scientific jargon to satisfy fantasies and cravings for the supernatural. It is a logical presentation of what the ancient yogis and its potential, and about how to harness that potential for our own betterment as well as for the elevation of humanity.

Chapter 1:

≈ All is Not What it Seems ≈

"Whatever you think, that you will be;
If you think yourself weak, weak you will be;
If you think yourself strong, strong you will be;
If you think yourself impure, impure you will be;
If you think yourself pure, pure you will be."
≈ Swami Vivekananda ≈

The Unseen Universe

There is an unseen aspect of the Universe, one that is imperceptible to our primary senses. It is the realm of subtle energies and forces fundamental to the creation and maintenance of the physical material world around us.

Ok, that's what the yogis tell us, anyhow. I think, though, that even the most skeptical person would still concede that there is probably something behind this entire visible, physical world that we move around in, even though they may not know what that "something" is or care to examine it any further at the moment.

According to the yogis, this "invisible realm," however one defines it, is influenced by human thought and emotions, and the forces within it react to those thoughts and emotions in distinct ways. Though the exact nature of thoughts and emotions may seem vague and intangible to most of us, never the less, those who have studied them know that they act upon the subtle, unseen reality as definite as magnetic force or electric current acts upon physical matter.

I know that the statement above can be a big pill to swallow. It is, after all, a subject that rarely gets explored much in mainstream science and education, and so it's reasonable to expect some skepticism. So right now, don't believe it if you don't want to. I'd like to ask you

though, to entertain the "basic idea" for the moment –
the notion that there is more to this existence than meets
the eye – and to stay with me here as I take you on a
deeper look into things through the eyes of the Yoga
scientists...

Our Untapped Potential

Everybody, regardless of race, religion, education, or
social or economic status, has an unlimited capacity of
"higher power" at their disposal – a capacity that is
inherent in their natural, inborn faculty of thought. It
would be convenient for me to point out at this time, the
fact that the average person uses only 10% of their brain's
capacity – convenience, except that it's simply not true
and I don't want to further propagate that myth. Yes,
experiments have shown that only around 10% of the
brain's neurons are typically active at any given time, but
which ones and in which areas of the brain depends on
what exactly the person is doing or thinking at the time.
The fact is that modern science doesn't know how much
of our brain is being used and if any of it remains unused
or underutilized at all. Capacity for complex thought and
how that capacity develops remains, for the most part, a
scientific mystery. All we really know right now, from a
modern scientific point of view, is that some people have
been able to develop greater intellectual capacities than
others, and that that development isn't necessarily a
reflection of their level of formal education.

Although the nature of "our thoughts" is something that
modern science has not yet been able to define to any
useful degree, the ancient yogic scientists seemed to have
found a way to understand this force, the way it works,
its effects, and its profound potential. More importantly,
they have shown us how to realize that potential.

3

Whether you look at things from a metaphysical or biological point of view, few would disagree that we are all tapping into only a fraction of our inherent mental potential. We're all still making use of some of our inherent capacity of thought to some degree or another. Typically though, it's on an unconscious level. That's not necessarily how we want to use our power of thought, because when we're operating on unconscious autopilot, so to speak, we're often causing more harm than good. We need to switch off that autopilot and take back the controls.

In order to become conscious of the potential of this great natural resource of ours and to use it productively and constructively, we need to start by exploring exactly what thought is, and how it works. I'm not going to break into a boring scientific paper – at least I'm going to try as best as I can not to, but we do have to cover a little bit of yogic science ground here, to get started.

Yoga Science 101

The yogis have a uniquely insightful way of viewing the phenomenon of thought, and admittedly, if you are new to Yoga, some of these ideas may take time to ponder and fully grasp. As best and as simply as I can, I'm going to take you on a guided journey through the yogic world view, step by step, so that by the end of this book you'll be able to understand what the ancient Rishis (Yogis) discovered and how to use that wisdom to transform your life in ways you might not even be able to imagine yet.

The Various Levels of Our Being

The basis for understanding thought lies in the yogic concept of the *pancha koshas* (five bodies). In Yoga, the human is conceived of as a multi-bodied being. These "bodies," or discernable aspects of man, differ in their essential nature, composition and function, and are arranged successively from the grosser, or more tangible, to the increasingly more subtle. They are:

1. ***Annamaya Kosha*** – This is the physical tissue or the cellular structure, referred to as the "physical sheath".
2. ***Pranamaya Kosha*** – Enveloping this grossest dimension of man is a more subtle body, the *pranamaya kosha*, "energy sheath." It is comprised of the vital energy known as *prana*, that which gives life to the otherwise lifeless physical body.
3. ***Manomaya Kosha*** – Encasing the *annamaya koshas* is yet another more subtle layer, that which is made up of conscious mind and memory, the "mental sheath" or *manomaya kosha.*
4. ***Vijnanamaya Kosha*** – The "sheath of intellect," it encloses the three lower bodies with what is sometimes also called the "super conscious mind," or *buddhi* (higher intellect).
5. ***Anandamaya Kosha*** – This is known as the body of "Cosmic Consciousness" or the "sheath of eternal bliss," which contains and envelops all the others.

Pancha Kosha - The Five Bodies of Man

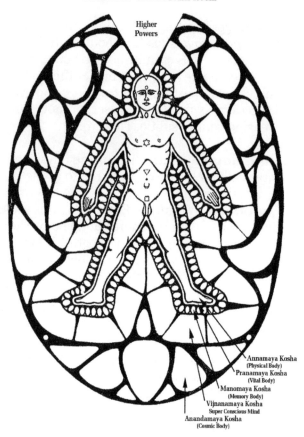

Higher
Powers

Annamaya Kosha
(Physical Body)
Pranamaya Kosha
(Vital Body)
Manomaya Kosha
(Memory Body)
Vijnanamaya Kosha
Super Conscious Mind
Anandamaya Kosha
(Cosmic Body)

Source: Yoga Step by Step

East Meets West on the Subatomic Level

Physicists have now substantiated that all matter and energy is essentially reducible to vibrations. This notion, at essence, helps to explain the concept of *energy* that lies at the heart of many traditions, "spiritual vocabulary." Though the concept of *energy* in new-age spirituality, which has now permeated well into mainstream culture, is often quite vague and rather ambiguous, in the science of Yoga these energies are precise and definite.

Everything from physical solids to energies such as heat, light and radiation oscillate, or vibrate, at different rates. All of these are scientifically measurable forces and perceivable, in one way or another, through the physical *annamaya kosha*. In Yoga, we recognize that it is within the more subtle bodies of the *pancha kosha* where the finer energies such as thought and awareness reside, an idea that might become a little more tangible as you read on.

Vibration

Once we grasp the way in which vibrations influence things, then we have the basis for understanding all energetic forces. Imagine a bumblebee that has fallen into a pool of water. The vibrations of its wings make tiny waves in the water, which in turn makes a leaf at the other end of the pool vibrate at exactly the same speed as the bee's wings.

Whenever anything vibrates, it sends these vibrations through the air (or makes the air itself vibrate). Depending on what is vibrating, the speed of these vibrations will vary. A drumhead, for instance, vibrates at a low speed sending big, slow waves through the air. A mosquito's wings vibrate very fast and will send tiny, fast waves vibrating through the air. We interpret vibrations of air as sound via the eardrum mechanism, a complicated set of bones and organs capable of interpreting vibrations as low as 20 vibrations per second (vps), or as high as 20,000 vps.

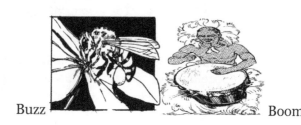

Buzz   Boom

Resonance and Our Response to Vibration

Yoga philosophy is based upon the idea that we are each a minute part of an infinite and inconceivable Universe. What happens in this vast Universe also has its counterpart in the physical world, our bodily selves included. This has been referred to in various ways in *Yoga*, such as macrocosm-microcosm, *purusha-prakrithi,* or *adhi-vyadhi.* The idea of attuning with various speeds of vibration, or coming into resonance with them then, is at the heart of much of Yoga's philosophy and practices.

Our individual response to the Universe occurs via the *principle of resonance.* Our body cells all respond, as modern science will attest, to vibrations of all levels. Our emotions and the subtle *pranic* (energy) field known as the *pranamaya kosha,* for instance, are influenced by

8

certain resonances, or speeds of vibrations that it comes into contact with. It is within the subtle matter of mental body, or *manomaya kosha* where thought activity resides. On these subtle plains we can observe the principle of resonance in play, the same as we observe it in scientific experiments in the physical world – for instance, as in the principle of sound resonance.

For example, a note on a string plucked on a musical instrument will set into vibration another string of that same note, which is tuned to the exact same pitch.

In this way, thought has the power and the potential, via this <u>principle of resonance</u>, to affect not only ourselves on many levels (mental, physical and emotional), but also our surrounding environment, including others within it.

Along with the "resonant effect", mental vibrations (thoughts) act in various other ways too, all following the principles of physics, just as light and sound does in the material world, to establish patterns, to generate force and to affect bodies, as I will be illustrating soon.

Man's Response to Vibrations

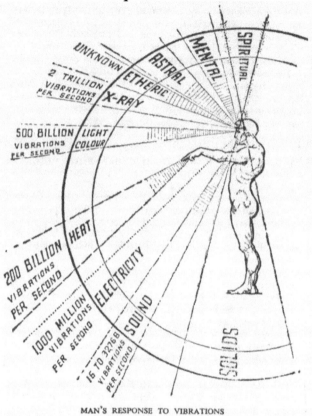

MAN'S RESPONSE TO VIBRATIONS

Source: Yoga Step by Step

Studies have found that humans respond in one way or another to various cosmic and earth-bound vibrational forces that come in contact with their mental, emotional and physical systems. In fact, the human organism acts like a bio-cosmic set of resonance forks, so to speak. Some vibrations can disturb the psychophysical harmony, whereas others can promote health, balance and wellbeing. These vibrations not only strongly influence the function of the organic organism, but it has become quite clear through modern scientific research that they also have a very powerful affect upon the electro-magnetic envelop of the body, or the *pranamaya kosha.*

Neurological science is also recognizing the effects of these energy vibrations upon the activity of the human brain. These discoveries, perhaps, will ultimately lead scientists into the metaphysical/para-physical realm of "higher vibrations' -- that mental and spiritual field which has always been the territory of the *raja yogi.*

Yoga itself is the science of resonance – of attuning oneself to the beneficial, evolutionary vibrations of the Universe. For instance, when certain vibrations produce relaxation of the nervous system, this enables the mind to freely concentrate upon the "inner reality." Conversely, vibrations that induce a state of stress and imbalance inhibit this ability.

This idea lies at the heart of many of our Yoga practices, such as *asana, kriya, mudra, pranayama,* and concentration *(dharana)* techniques.

Chapter 2:

≈ The Power of Thought ≈

"Healing, Manifesting and Transforming
Through Yoga"

≈ Yogacharya ≈

The Thought Effect

You may have never considered where your thoughts come from or what role you've actually had in creating them. You might even think that your thoughts are things that just happen on their own – ideas that appear from "somewhere" and just flow through your head – and that there is not much you can do about them. But if we stop for a second to think about that, it's obviously not true. I guess the act of stopping for a second to think about it is all we need to do to really prove that point – the point that we actually do decide what flows through our heads – at least when we want to. Hopefully, by the end of this book, you'll have more than enough reasons to want to take back a little control over that sea of mental activity swirling through your noggin all day, and also have a bit of an idea of how to do it.

In the previous chapter we laid a basic framework of the nature of thought from a yogic perspective. I know that for some folks those ideas may be pretty unfamiliar, so it's okay if you're still finding all this a bit tough to swallow. In this chapter we will look at some more tangible, real-world examples that should help it all start to make some sense. We're not quite finished with the Yoga science class yet though!

How Thought Affects Us

If we were to examine what factors are involved in creating every state of health we could possibly experience, be it good or bad, it's unlikely that thought would not be a part of the equation every time. There are only two basic ways though, that thought affects our health and wellbeing, and to illustrate them I'm going to start by building a little further upon the yogic idea of the *pancha koshas* (five bodies).

The biggest personal impact our thoughts have is directly upon our mental body (*manomaya kosha*), establishing what the yogis call *samskaras*. *Samskaras* are patterns or conditioned responses that have become ingrained within our subconscious over time, simply as a result of repetition. These patterns are established one after the other throughout our lifetime of experiences and actions, and by the time we are fully functioning, independently thinking adults, and our mental body is chalked full of them. The irony, I suppose, is that we actually aren't really as "independently thinking" as we might believe ourselves to be. Most of what we think, and the vast majority of our opinions and evaluations of situations are based upon deeply-rooted subconscious beliefs – specific ways that we've become used to viewing things that may or may not be as well-founded as we think.

In simple terms, *samskaras* work like this: Each subconscious pattern consists of its own unique "rate of oscillation," or vibration within the mental body. The "mind," gets accustomed to these vibrations, or "patterns of thought," and tends to return to them as soon as possible whenever it has been forced away by some other new or less accustomed thought or feeling. Ok, that may sound a tad scientific, but surely we can all relate to that idea. How easy is it to remember your ten-times tables, and how hard is it to wrap your head around organic chemistry, for instance? One you learned when you were 6 years old, and have been performing over and over again automatically for years ... and the other you just tried to get a passing grade in to fulfill your science credits to graduate, and then never gave it another thought after that.

But what if you suddenly found out that ten times ten was not 100? What if it was 99? I mean, did you ever make 10 piles of apples and then put them all together and count to make sure there were 100 apples in the pile?

Ok, let me save you the trouble. I did, and ten times ten does indeed equal 100 (surprise!). But if it didn't, I'm sure I would have a real uphill battle trying to convince you to believe it, wouldn't I?

The point here is not about questioning the validity of algebra. The point I'm trying to make, and I hope I did, is that the more one experiences a particular thought or emotion, the more predominant, or established (rooted) its vibrational pattern becomes within the mind (mental body), and the harder it is to change it.

Old Habits Are Hard to Break

What if we didn't have this pre-programmable personal hard drive, so to speak? What a pain it would be to have to sit down with a pen and paper to figure out if you have enough money in your wallet to pay for the groceries you just bought. So *samskaras* aren't necessarily bad. They are Nature's way of helping us to function more efficiently through life.

The problem is with the innumerable ways that we've come to see and perceive things. The countless ideas and concepts that we've come to accept as "true"; all the things that we base our entire way of viewing this world and everything in it, which have all been laid down, over time firmly within our subconscious. A lot of these things may not be quite as easily verifiable as your ten-times tables, but most of them you have come to accept just as firmly (subconsciously) as being true.

To a certain extent we're all afflicted with this sort of "virtual reality" belief structure. It's part and parcel of the nature of life, where a great deal of what we believe to be true is probably only partially true, while some of what we believe may even be down right false!

No, you haven't been duped. This simply happens because we've been conditioned by all of our external influences: our teachers, our neighbors, our cultures, our religions and our mass media to see things a certain way. The thing is that most of those who were playing these heavily influential roles in our lives were in fact, unknowingly operating on a lot of their own incorrect assumptions and partial truths – which is why they were able to pass them on to you so convincingly. You can probably see how "reality" can easily become elusive in an environment like that.

That sort of seems a bit depressing, doesn't it? Or maybe alarming is a better word? Well relax. I don't want to thrust you into an existential crisis here (not yet anyhow, we're only on page 13). My simple aim at this stage is just to ask you to consider that some of the things you believe may not quite be as cut and dry as you thought – that's all.

So let's assume, for a moment, that some of the things we thought we knew all about aren't quite as they seem.

16

How is it that we aren't able to simply see that? Or rather, why is it often so hard for us to change our views about something?

The Law of "Repetition Creates Tendency" (or something like that, anyhow...)

There is a reason why it's "hard to teach an old dog new tricks," as the saying goes. The stronger a thought (or belief), the greater influence or effect that it has on all the vibrations within the mental body as a whole, essentially persuading all the vibrations within the entire "mental sheath" to move at this same rate. Maybe that sounds a little too scientific to be coming from the mouths of the ancient yogis, but if they were here now and well versed in the lingo of the modern technical age, something like that is probably what they would say.

What they did discover long ago, though, is that every time a thought is repeated it is a little easier for the same thought to happen again. A habit of vibrating at that particular rate is being set up in the mental body, which causes a tendency for that exact thought to be repeated when another opportunity arises.

Surely we can all relate to this principle? How many times have you, in frustration with a friend or family member, started a sentence with, "You always do (this ...)" or "Why can't you ever do (that ...)?"

We all know that in reality nobody ever "always does something." But in your mind you've decided that they do, and when that annoying behavior of theirs pops up and you are gripped by an instant of high emotion, you instinctively react with this wrong view of them that has been conditioned in your little head as being "a fact."

What about another example that does not involve such highly charged emotion? Let's say you are a meat eater. You obviously see this as perfectly natural and normal and nothing to really view as out of the ordinary. However, eating insects, to you, may be disgusting and repulsive. Then you travel to Thailand and find you are strolling through the night market in Bangkok with stalls upon stalls of people cooking and munching happily away on various roaches on a stick! EWE! That Thai person feels exactly the same way about larvae and grasshoppers that you do about a roast beef sandwich. In other words, "what's so strange about eating bugs?"

A logical, detached mind would see absolutely no difference between the two. So wherein lays the facts? Which belief (bug eater or beef eater) merely reflects the way we've been conditioned to view "real food." Which one really is a repulsive eating habit? Neither? Both?

The yogis do have a definite philosophy about diet and nutrition, and I'm not going to delve into that in this book. This example is just an easily tangible way for most of us to start to take notice that our attitudes and beliefs are not always based upon any real, unquestionable facts. Rather, they are quite often based simply upon the way that we've come to see things as a result of, among other things, our cultural conditioning – what the people where we come from do, and what we've been taught by our parents as a result. In other words, it's (almost) all in your head!

Taking Advantage of Our Mental Tendencies

I hope that you're still holding that existential crisis at bay. I say that in jest, but in reality, realizing that a lot of what forms our foundation of ideas and beliefs is just stuff that was unwittingly planted inside our heads and is not necessarily based upon any Universal truths, it can definitely be disturbing at first. But this is not about spreading doom and gloom. In fact, it's just the opposite. It presents a great opportunity for positive, productive change. Of course, change usually requires some shifts that may, initially, feel a bit uncomfortable. Once we've allowed ourselves to make that move, we might discover that the view where we end up is a lot better.

The principle that *repetition creates tendency,* may mean that many of our current beliefs and ideas are only somewhat true, or in some cases even way off the mark. It also explains why negative emotions and opinions are so hard to break free from and end up being extremely detrimental to our health and wellbeing. The same principle also has a bright side. It illustrates the power that "positive thinking" can have on adjusting those *samskaras,* those conditioned mental habits and responses. In fact, many practices in Yoga are designed to do exactly that – to replace old, relentlessly negative (or lower) thoughts with persistent new ones of a more positive, healthier nature.

"I Think, Therefore I Obsess"

Obsession isn't just a fragrance by Calvin Klein – it's a crippling part of the human psyche. In many ways, it's the most detrimental mental disease, not only because it hampers one's ability to think rationally and objectively, but also because it affects nearly everyone today to some degree or another.

With the previously outlined yogic views in mind, it's easy to work out how mental fixations are created. Obsessions are thoughts that, when repeated often enough with a certain strength, become almost automatic, or pathological in their consistency. To follow along with our more scientific explanation from earlier, the vibration becomes so strong that it overrides almost all other "mental activity" within the mental body, to the point where one can't or doesn't want to change how they are thinking and feeling – they are mentally consumed with one thing and one thing only.

This "mental rut" can occur when a recurring thought is of a specific nature, with its focus on a particular thing – perhaps a desire or want, a sexual obsession, or even something so simple as feeling the need to have a piece of chocolate cake RIGHT NOW! Yeah, when you're cranky as a boar until you've had your morning coffee, you know what I'm talking about here.

We don't' have to know exactly what we're fixated upon, to still fall into this same kind of obsessive mental rut. It can also occur when the "general theme of recurring thought" is of one type or another, for instance, of a positive or negative, or happy or sad nature. That's why happy people tend to want to hang out with happy people and do fun things all the time and also why "misery loves company."

So obviously it works both ways. These types of mental fixations can just as easily bring us up, as they can hold us down. But is one good and the other bad, necessarily?

Remember, we're talking about striving to rise above our subconscious conditionings for a reason. The whole premise around seeking to see things as they "are", and not as "we've come to believe them to be" is that we think this clarity will ultimately bring us to a place of better health and wellbeing. From the perspective of the yogis, the goal is to take us even farther than that – to a more evolved, spiritually enlightened state of mind, so to speak.

One of my favorite passages comes from the ancient Katha Upanishad, which states, "Don't mistake the pleasant for the good. That which is pleasant is not always good for us and that which is good for us is not always pleasant." With that piece of wisdom in mind, it's clear that simply obsessing in thoughts that may feel nice at the time, but still be based upon some level of fantasy, will always hold us back from the highest joy that can only be known by ridding ourselves of ALL our delusions. As you might have guessed; however, being able to tell the difference may not be as easy as it sounds.

Many people confuse romance with love – or rather, they confuse the euphoric feelings of being desired by another and being showered with attention and tenderness with what love really means. Real love is not based upon something as superficial as physical attraction; nor is it dependent upon receiving any of that same kind of admiration in return. Love is the highest of emotions that many who utter the word may have not ever really experienced it. Love is the willingness to put another's best interests above one's own. It is the willingness to help another to face the root causes of their troubles, even if that means facing unpleasant truths and difficult circumstances; and it is a willingness to be their unmovable rock of support through that often unpleasant process, without expectation or desire for anything in return. And just in case you are still wondering – no, love has absolutely nothing to do with diamond rings!

We often see this same idea at work in new-age spirituality, where the pursuit of feeling good is often mistaken for the guiding light toward a more evolved life. We have to be careful about falling into this trap, and

21

that sometimes these feelings are nothing more than another security blanket that keeps us from learning the lessons we are all put upon this earth to learn, in order to truly grow and evolve.

Rising Out of the Swamp of Negativity

I bring up the idea of being deluded by so-called happy feelings because, in many ways, that is the more dangerous state of mind to be in – more dangerous because it's easy to think that everything is well and good. On the flip side, things seem a little more obvious. It can be particularly destructive for someone when almost all of his or her thoughts are of a generally negative nature. If that state of mind is allowed to remain too long, it can ultimately lead to an inability to rise above negative thoughts at all.

This seems to be a state of mind that is becoming more and more common now, as disenchantment; feelings of helplessness, futility and depression continue to rise. It's probably not too much of a stretch to suggest that modern lifestyles have had a lot to do with this unfortunate reality today. As societies, we are certainly becoming more and more disconnected from nature, while our foundations are no longer rooted in higher spiritual, holistic values, like they perhaps were more so in historical times.

A concept know as *pratipaksha bhavana,* to counter this disparaging possibility, is still rooted deep within Indian culture, whereby when a negative or disturbing thought, emotion, situation or event occurs; one makes a conscious effort to cultivate the opposite, more virtuous and positive attitude and response. To a Westerner, on the surface this may seem like a peculiar, even weak-willed habit of always trying to be nice or wanting to avoid conflict, which can even frustrate the seemingly manic Westerner to want dissent and confrontation. But the ancients of the Indian Subcontinent well understood the power of thought and, as I mentioned earlier, through the ages interwove this so-called, well-mannered behavior into the fabric of their culture. That cultural protocol served, as it still does to a certain extent today, as a means to avoid the creation of negative *samskaras*, as well as to break down existing negative patterns within the subconscious mind – and to transplant upon the fertile ground a foundation of virtue and goodness.

Carpé Diem

Pratipaksha bhavana, although it may seem like a rather simple, ineffectual concept, is actually quite an astounding practice. Students whom I have directed through this process have reported back with surprising delight at how transformative it has been for them, both in terms of their own mindset, as well as with the positive effects it has yielded in their interactions with others. From my own personal experiments, I would agree that this practice definitely leads to more than one might have expected.

If you're attempting to experiment for the first time with this concept, then there are a couple guidelines in order for it to really work. With *pratipaksha bhavana,* it's imperative to act immediately, upon the first inklings of awareness, right at the conception of "negativity," before the vibration of that negative establishes itself with any firmness within the mind. It is also important to remember that the greater the emotion attached to a thought, the more powerful the thought (vibration) is. So, in *pratipaksha bvanana* one should replace the harmful thought with a strong, emotion-laden one of a more virtuous and positive nature.

Remember, as we think, so shall we act, and in action so shall habit form. Therefore, like anything, trying it once won't really do anything for you – not any more than, say, eating a carrot once, and then going back to your steady diet of burgers and ice cream. It's in the constant repetition of this action of "taking the opposite view" that mental transformation ultimately will happen. A Hindu/Buddhist axiom goes as follows:

"Sow a thought, reap an action, sow an action, reap a habit, sow a habit, reap a characteristic, sow a characteristic, and reap a destiny!"

In that one profound, simple saying, the authority of thought over one's personal destiny is plain as pie.

Out of the Mind and Into the Body

In a nutshell, the previous chapter illustrated the primary effect that thought has upon us, which is laying down *samskaras* – patterns or conditioned ways of thinking and acting – into our subconscious mind, at the level of the mental body or *manomaya kosha*.

There is a second effect that thought has upon us though, and it is equally as important. It's the effect that it has on the adjacent bodies above and below the *manomaya kosha*. Recall that these bodies are the *vijnanamaya kosha*, the "super conscious mind," and *anandamaya kosha*, the "cosmic body," which are the more subtle sheaths above; and the denser *pranamaya kosha*, the emotional/energy body and *annamaya kosha*, the physical body below.

24

As in the physical world, activity in one form of matter can readily affect another form. In the physical world, for instance, an earthquake can produce a mighty wave in the sea above it, while the movement of the air, depending on its intensity, will produce ripples or even great waves in the ocean beneath it. So in the same way, activity in one's "mental body" will affect these other adjacent levels of their being too. In practical terms, that means thought can elicit emotional responses by affecting the *pranamaya kosha,* the emotional body directly adjacent to it while, conversely, emotions can affect how we think. In other words, our emotions can create patterns in the way we think, react, and view things. Remember the "You always do this!" example from earlier?

Emotions, in turn, will affect their adjacent physical structure, the *annamaya kosha,* in various positive or negative ways. Do you hold stress in your shoulders? Now you know why. Actually, that's probably not news to many of us any more – that our emotions lead to a whole host of physical manifestations, both good and bad. Medical science has its own way of explaining this mind/body relationship via the stress-response mechanisms and the glandular/hormonal systems and their response to various emotional states. It is interesting to see that the ancient Yoga scientists, hundreds of years before the human body was dissected and examined under a microscope, had such a precise understanding of this causal relationship too. Perhaps even more importantly, they figured out exactly what to do about it.

We'll tread that ground a bit later on, but for now, you can see that the power of thought to affect our physical condition resides in our ability to properly control our emotions. I don't want you to misread that statement

25

though. I said, "properly control," not "suppress." There's a big difference, but we'll get to that later as well.

Thinking of evolving?

In the opposite direction, the directions of greater subtlety "above" the mental body – *vijnanamaya kosha* (the super conscious mind) and *anandamaya kosha* (the cosmic body), our habitual thought patterns have the potential to elevate our consciousness. There's a flip side to every coin though, and you guessed it, our thoughts also have as much potential to hold us back on that evolutionary road.

This talk about evolution needs a bit of a backdrop because that word means different things to different people. A brief outline of the yogic view of reality will help get us all on the same page.

Chapter 3:

≈ The Yogic View of Reality ≈

The Yogic View of Reality

People interested in Yoga today come from a variety of cultural and religious backgrounds, which means that many of the yogic concepts, like some of those I've introduced to you so far, can be pretty unfamiliar, or even totally perplexing to some folks. So if you're having a hard time wrapping your head around some of this stuff so far, you can bet you're not alone. At least you're still reading, which is good because I think things will start to feel a bit more "real" to you soon. What we need to do first though, to put all of this into a more solid content, is take a step back and have a quick look at where the ancient yogis are coming from – what their basic view of "reality" is, and why they see things the way they do.

The Science of Truth

All scientists have one thing in common – their quest for the truth. Though their methods may have differed from those of today's scientists, the ancient Yoga scientists had that same primary goal – to know the unknown and to remove ignorance through greater understanding. Over generations of their experiments with truth, the Yoga Rishis gained a unique understanding of the nature of the Universe and our place as human beings within it. The worldview that they were able to outline, as a result, is so comprehensive that its framework continues to support, time and time again, new discoveries in all fields of science and medicine. The findings of Yoga are every bit as logical and verifiable as those of modern science, though few today have really taken the time to properly examine this ancient science to find out what it's really all about – preferring instead to brush Yoga aside with little regard, or portray it most inaccurately as a religion of sorts.

Those; however, who have taken the time to properly explore Yoga, understand why it is called "The Science of Truth," and also often referred to as "The Science of all Sciences." They know that Yoga is the means by which to uncover the ultimate reality that sits veiled behind the bias of all-external, humanly influences – like cultural attitudes, religious rhetoric and especially the narrow constraints of modern scientific thought, which have yet to be overcome.

The Science of Yoga could also aptly be called the "Science of First-hand Experience," because although its teachings often contain poetic, metaphorical and symbolic language used to paint broad landscapes of perception and ideas, its wisdom and understanding relies ultimately upon genuine experience – experience which is gained through a comprehensive, graduated system of practices designed to lead to body and mind through successively greater stages of awareness and understanding.

"Self-knowledge is not attained by someone who is not introspective. Thus scripture [Katha-Upanishad 1.2.22] states: 'This Self is not attained by discussion, intelligence, or learning.'"
≈ Jivanmukti-Viveka ≈

29

The Nature of Reality

The Eastern world-view is based upon the idea of the "unity of all things," and is reflected in the spiritual traditions of Hinduism, Buddhism, Taoism, and also Yoga. If you've studied Yoga or Eastern philosophy at all, then you may have heard the term "non-dualism," which denotes this fundamental belief. Non-dualism means that we cannot speak of God without speaking of man, nor speak of man, without speaking of God, because they are one and the same – inseparable at their essence. It means that there is no actual separate "self," no "you" or "I" to speak of – that we, along with everything that is seen or unseen in this vast universe, are all just minute parts of one, unified and divine source.

The Unity of All Things

Unity, the ultimate, indivisible reality, known as the "Tao" in Taoism, as *Dharmakaya* or *Tathata* in Buddhism, is referred to as *Brahman* in Hinduism – the *Unitive Principle,* or the indivisible *One Reality,* which manifests in all things. The word Yoga comes from the Sanskrit root *yuj,* meaning "to join" or "unite," revealing that the real goal of Yoga is certainly a lofty one. Yoga is, in fact, a science designed to ultimately take us beyond this perception of separateness that we have, this idea that we are something unique and individual, to the ultimate realization of that *oneness,* a state referred to in Yoga as *Samadhi.*

Oneness
By: Meenakshi Devi Bhavanani

Everyone wants oneness in some form or another. The unitive impulse is deeply imbedded in our DNA. But everyone seeks that union in a different way, and according to their own level of consciousness ... none of us likes the sense of the presence of "the other." When we sense *otherness*, we instinctively try to remove it in various ways according to our level of evolution. At the lower animal level, we can remove the sense of the otherness by killing it, eating it, mating with it, or chasing it away.

This kind of *oneness* is still practiced by man, Homo erectus, who is still mostly dominated by his animal brain. Perhaps 90% of the human race still exists on this level of consciousness and this is one explanation for the horrendous wars and conflicts, which are ravaging the earth. "There should be *only one*, and the *only one* should be *me,*" thinks the animal brain. This is a very crude concept of oneness.

The egotistical man, who has risen above herd consciousness and above mob allegiances, interprets this primordial urge for oneness in more subtle ways. He may no longer kill, eat, mate with or chase away *the other,* but he will try to submerge the other in his own ego presence. This can be done through social, political, emotional or economic dominance. He thus creates the presence of *one will* or *one aim,* which dominate *the other* ... Charismatic leaders such as Napoleon, Hitler, Mussolini, Stalin, Franco and Moa all demonstrated this kind of *oneness* ... Of course; history shows us clearly where all those crude attempts at oneness end.

... As one rises in evolution though, one chooses more refined methods of achieving oneness and erasing the sense of otherness. ... This may be expressed in a more refined sense such as sports, competitions, take over bids in business, different kinds of national and international gatherings that seek to resolve the *otherness* through various methods of communication and communion, through conferences, political parties, rallies, etc. Even the frenzied gatherings inspired by rock stars are an attempt of the masses to experience a primordial and still crude kind of oneness.

... Some think that they can banish that terrifying sense of *otherness* by finding the perfect mate. The man and woman unite and create the child and *one unit* is formed ... [But] sooner or later even this family unit has to brush up against *the other*, and the [same] old patterns emerge. ... Emotional bonds are formed to create a oneness, but emotions are fickle and unstable. That kind of oneness can only be transient.

... Those forces, which push us toward union, are powerful and strong. Perhaps the Universe is saying, "Look! Sooner or later you have to come back to me. What you are looking for here and there can only be found in the Real, True and Permanent sense, when you lift your eyes to the sky and realize that *all is in essence, oneness.*" ... At the top of the evolutionary ladder, at the peak, the point, the tip of the mountain, there is only *oneness*. It is to those heights that this primordial unitive impulse seeks to propel us. The journey up this big and treacherous mountain may take us thousands of lifetimes, but it is a journey that we all have to make ... sooner or later. But, as the Guru says, "if not now, when?"

The Ego Self

The concept of the *ego self* is a fundamental one in Yoga philosophy. I have noticed that this use of the word *ego;* however, sometimes evokes a particular type of defensiveness in those from Western cultures, where it has somewhat different connotations. The *ego,* though, has a very profound place within Eastern thought and its proper understanding is essential to the interpretation of much of the teachings of Yoga.

In Western culture, the word *ego* is usually associated with arrogance, selfishness, inflated self-importance, and an unjustified feeling of superiority. It has come to refer to a certain characteristic of an individual that makes them rather unpleasant and often intolerable in the eyes of others. Though in Yoga we certainly would not disagree with those descriptions, we also understand that those notions represent only the grossest inflation of the *ego*.

The *ego* that the yogis speak of is the sense of "I" which we *all* possess. "I have this...," "I am that...," I do this...," "I like that...," "I feel," "I eat," "I sleep," etc., etc. The *ego* is that sense of being a separate, thinking, feeling, sleeping, eating, doing human being, which is in itself a result of our dualistic perception of reality – of our loss of the sense of *oneness*. This ego-state is referred to in Yoga as the "I Consciousness," or more commonly, "the *ego self.*"

Having an *ego* is not necessarily a bad thing. In fact, it is part and parcel of our existence in this material world. The yogis point out to us; however, that this *ego* is not actually real. It is not the truth of our nature. It is a concept that exists purely in our dualistic-thinking minds, and is nowhere else to be found.

An Illusionary Life

Don't confuse self-confidence with arrogance. The yogi is self-confident. He (or she) knows that what he says is true because he has done the necessary exploration to know what the Truth is. But he does not crave recognition, appreciation, or any special credit because of it. Contrast that with the typical person whose sense of worth is defined by their importance in the eyes of others, and whose life is spent continuously striving to inflate his/her self-importance. This is what we all do, although we may not even realize it. We are motivated by our achievements, by our awards and our certificates, by our successes in business, by our ability to gain the love and affections of others, by our stature in the communities and even our standing within our families. We may think that we are altruistic in our ways, doing what we do for the betterment of humanity, but few are as noble as they envision themselves to be. When it comes right down to it, we all still see ourselves as real, separate, isolated beings with our own needs, our own ability to act independently and our own ability to possess. The greater this feeling of "I" that we have, the further separation in the mind from the sense of oneness we have – the greater our ignorance of the *True Self*.

Transcending the Ego

The *True Self,* that essence of our being that underlies our surface image, or ego, can still proceed effectively in worldly affairs and achieve whatever we set out to do. Yet, by being able to proceed with that greater awareness, we won't be motivated by selfish gain. Instead, we'll make decisions that are for the greater good of humanity and not the good of the "I" alone. Power, influence, wealth and material affluence can just as readily come to one who has risen above the sense of "me" and "mine," yet this power and wealth does not stimulate conceit, superiority or vanity. Rather, it stimulates a sense of reverence, gratitude and duty toward fellow human beings and all of creation.

"The sage centered in the Self should think, 'I do nothing at all' – though seeing, hearing, touching, smelling, eating, going, sleeping, breathing, speaking, emptying, holding, opening and closing the eyes – firm in the thought that the senses move among sense object."
≈ Bhagavad Gita (Chapter 5, Verse 11) ≈

When we transcend the *ego,* that sense of separation and duality, then we have regained the send of *oneness.* This is really what the word *enlightenment* refers to. But in transcending the *ego,* we're speaking here of the highest ideal. For the vast majority of people on the earth today, this "total realization" will likely escape them throughout their current lifetime. This doesn't mean that we all cannot and will not find immense value in our lives and in our spiritual pursuits. In fact, we can and we will! We will all evolve at our own pace, life after life, knowing that the highest ideal is our unavoidable destiny!

The understanding of the *ego* holds the key to a vastness of human potential; be in leading a more holistic and naturally aware life; finding health, peace and harmony, experiencing all of life with the utmost sense of joy; or basking in the contentment and sense of fulfillment that wisdom and truth bestows. These attainments are all inversely proportionate to the *ego self.* As we lessen the *ego,* we gain in spirit; but as we build up and protect the *ego* to further degrees, we lose our ability to truly experience any of these wonderful things.

The Unfolding of the Universe

All the world's a stage,
And all the men and women merely players;
They have their exits and their entrances,
And one man in his time plays many parts ...
≈ William Shakespeare (*As You Like It 2/7*) ≈

An Upanishad (ancient Indian scripture) says, "That which was one became the many." The basic recurring theme in Indian mythology is the creation of the world by the self-sacrifice of the Supreme "God" – in the original meaning of the word "to make sacred" – whereby God becomes the world, which in the end, returns to God again. This creative activity of the Diving is called *Lila,* the *Play of God,* and the world, or manifest Universe, is seen as the stage of the Divine play.

Current belief in the science of astronomy is that the creation of the Universe, its growth, its eventual decay and regeneration are eternal processes without a beginning and without an end, repeating in endless cycles. In Hinduism, one full cycle of this creation and dissolution is known as a "day and night of *Brahman*." Indian mythology illustrates this universal cycle with *Brahman* as the Supreme Creator who transforms himself into the world with his mighty creative power. The word *maya* signifies this *might* or *power*. Commonly *maya* is defined as "illusion," referring to the mental state of anyone who is caught under the spell of *Lila,* or the Divine, cosmic play. As long as one continues to confuse the multitude of forms in this Divine play with *reality*, without perceiving the unity of *Brahman* underlying all of these forms, then they are said to be under the spell of the illusion *(maya). Maya,* therefore, does not mean that "the world is an illusion," as is often misleadingly stated. *Maya* is the illusion of mistaking the concepts of our mind – its measuring and categorizing of the myriad of forms of the Divine play – for reality of confusing the map with the territory, so to speak.

The Journey of the Jiva

Western philosophers have long grappled with the question, "What is the meaning of Life?" The underlying ambition of Eastern life, exemplified in a myriad of tales, legends and myths, reveals the answer to this question plainly to the Eastern spiritualist. It is the age-old expedition from darkness to the light, from ignorance to understanding. It is the quest for Self-realization. The meaning and highest purpose of life is simply the return of the "many to the One," the re-union of the *jiva,* the individual soul, with *Paramatman,* the eternal source.

Yet it is upon the stage of this timeless cosmic drama *(Lila)*, and under the spell of *maya* where that heroic voyage takes place. Beneath this veil from reality – our forgetting of the unity of *Brahman* – a sense of duality *(dwaitam)*, a sense of separateness emerges. This is the *ego-self,* the sense of a self that is unique and separate from others and the surrounding world. Self-realization, then, is merely in the re-realization of the true state of *oneness* -- the *reunion* of the individual with the universal. This is referred to various times in Yoga as *moksha, Samadhi, kaivalya,* or *jivana mukta,* the goal of Yoga and by all Eastern philosophical and spiritual accounts, the true meaning and purpose of life.

The Garuda Purana (an ancient Indian scripture) states that the long evolutionary journey of the *jiva* to its reunion with *Paramatman,* or Universal Soul, takes 84 lakhs (8.4 million) incarnations. Whether literal or figurative, it is a long process. At the same time; however, we're reminded that it's the natural, unconscious destiny of the "many" to return to the "One." The long, evolutionary process is what Yoga endeavors to consciously accelerate – hence, we also refer to the science of Yoga as "the Science of Conscious Evolution."

This is also why many Eastern spiritual cultures do not view death as a tragedy or as an end. Death is simply seen as a natural necessity in the process of evolution, as a continual transition along the evolutionary path of the Soul on its way back to God. A poem by Rumi, the great Sufi mystic, illustrates this sentiment beautifully:

> I died as a mineral to become a plant
> I died as a plant to become an animal
> I died as an animal to become a human
> I died as a human to become an angel
> I died as an angel to become a God
> When was I ever the lesser for dying?"

So this process of the unfolding and expansion of the consciousness back to the ultimate state of Self-realization is the evolutionary process we speak of in Yoga. When we speak in Yoga of leading an evolutionary life, we are talking about living here and now in this world, experiencing all of the good and the bad, and the ups and the downs, while at the same time, never losing site that there is a greater depth to this person we call "our self". One that is not dependent upon the achievements of this world for anything meaningful; and one that does not exist in contrast or conflict with others or the surrounding world, but in harmony with them. An evolutionary life is a life in which the certainty of this realization continues to steadily grow, while at the same time the turmoil of the world and its influence upon us gradually diminishes.

Evolutionary Thought

In the chapter previous to this one, we touched a little bit upon the idea of *evolutionary thought*. Now, with this short introduction to the yogic view of reality, that notion should have a little more contexts. The long and short of it is that thought has equal bearing upon both our emotional and physical health, as well as upon the level of our so-called "spiritual state" – our ability to separate ourselves from the delusion that we are this *ego self* that we've come to know and love so much, and move toward a higher state of understanding of our innate, unified nature.

Chapter 4:

≈ Healthy Thinking ≈

Healthy Thinking

In Chapter 2, I illustrated that a thought might be confined to the field of the mental body or it might affect any of the levels (*koshas*) above or below it. How exactly, depends upon the nature of the thought. For instance, thoughts of an intellectual nature, like a mathematical problem, will mainly affect the mental matter and remain for the most part restricted to the *manomaya kosha*, the mental sheath. If a thought is tainted with selfish desire, delusion or greed, its oscillations draw downward, expending most of their force with the emotional body, or *pranamaya kosha*, manifesting as well in the lower physical body, *annamaya kosha*, to one degree or another as tension, stress, disease, etc.

Conversely, if a thought is of a pure, or higher spiritual nature – a concept referred to as *sattvic* in the Sanskrit language – such as a profound sense of love or feeling of selflessness, it will rise upwards into the realm of the higher intellect, revealing a great power for evolution and personal transformation.

That much, we've already touched upon. We can easily see this in action. A person who is consumed with thoughts of a selfish nature frequently displays negative emotional states such as fear, anxiety, distrust, unfriendliness, etc., and usually has corresponding tension and ill-health within their physical body. Whereas, someone who is selfless, caring and

41

compassionate in mindset is also joyful, optimistic, confident, content, emotionally stable, and more often physically healthy. Wow! Who knew it was that easy to be healthy? Just change the way you think!

I "Think" I'm Healthy

Yes, thought plays an extremely important role in the state of our physical health. Consider the man who went to the doctor in a frantic state.

"What is the problem?" asked the doctor.
"I don't know," said the man. "I'm going crazy with anxiety here. My mind is bouncing back and forth and back and forth. One minute I think that I'm a tepee, the next minute I think that I'm a wigwam!"
"Ahh," replied the doctor with comforting relief in his voice. "Don't worry. I know exactly what the problem is. You're just two tents!"

This is all-to-often the problem, isn't it? The modern mind flip-flops from one ridiculous thought to another, all the while creating a vicious cycle of mental "tent-sion" that inhibits our ability to control even our own mental environment. The various meditation traditions refer to this similarly as "the monkey mind." In the Yoga Sutras (a classic yoga text), the great Sage Patanjali refers to this as *chitta vritti,* or "whirlpools of the mind." This mental restlessness or tension reverberates down through the *Pranamaya Kosha*, establishing disturbing patterns of emotions, which in turn manifest within the physical structure (*manomaya kosha)* in a whole host of modern day stress-related diseases.

Thought then, possesses enormous power to affect the current state of our physical body. Since this type of effect manifests most strongly from "subtle to gross," the state of our physical health results ultimately from our state of mind, which parallels the Western concept of psychosomatics. With this principle, we can even go so far as to suggest that all physical body manifestations result from activity originating at a higher *kosha* level, namely the *manomaya* and *pranamaya kosha,* the mental and emotional bodies respectively. Much of what manifest in the physical body results from either conscious or unconscious "mentalizations." These mentalizations can be ingrained beliefs, past traumas, conditioned patterns (*samskaras*), insecurities, projections, desires, delusions, attachments, etc.. all combining in force to ultimately build the state of our physical body as well as to inflict disturbances and diseases upon it.

The yogis have told us what many modern spiritualists also acknowledge – that by overcoming these types of damaging mental activities we can cure any and all that ails us on a physical level. Still much to the bewilderment of the modern medical world, the ability to cure oneself of physical disease through the mind has been demonstrated time and time again: a terminally diagnosed cancer patient miraculously recovers; a patient with a spinal injury who was told by their doctors that they'd never walk again, somehow does; tumors shrink, sensations return to nerve damaged limbs, lost site and hearing comes back. We hear of these kinds of things happening all the time, and the only real response that the medical community has when this happens is to shrug their shoulders and say, "Well, we have no idea why."

Even though the mechanisms of action are still not fully understood by the Western medical establishment, increasing investigation by the orthodoxy into the relationship between body, mind and emotions is revealing what the yogis have known for millennia – the immense power of the mind to affect the health and healing of the body. For example, a recent study in Europe (1) concluded that the most optimistic among a group of 545 men had a roughly 50% lower risk of cardiovascular death. The same study also notes, *"previous research has suggested that being optimistic boosts overall health and lowers the risk of death from all causes,"* and that *"a positive attitude also has been shown to help patients who suffer from heart disease."*

There is, in fact, a fair amount of research that supports the idea that mental attitudes do contribute measurably to physical health. For instance, several studies centered around a positive attitude showed that optimism leads to lower rates of re-hospitalization after heart surgery (2), protects against coronary heart disease in older men (3), and lowers the risk of stroke (4). Similar results were found in studies specifically targeting women. One concluded that higher levels of optimism at the start of chemotherapy reduced the levels of ovarian cancer antigens during treatment (5). Another found that optimism yielded lower cancer related as well as coronary heart disease related mortality, while cynical hostility had the exact opposite effect (6).

Along those same lines, studies concerning several different diseases have found that those who maintain positive feelings of well-being have a better survival rate (7). A Canadian-based study also observed that happiness and positive attitude reduced 10-years incident coronary heart disease (8), while another revealed a direct correlation between psychological well-being and a slower decline of health in old age (9). Positive emotions in general were also found to lower blood pressure in the elderly (10).

Research on the flip side suggests that negative emotions definitely have a detrimental effect on health. Chronic anger and hostility, along with neuroticism were found to be the biggest risk factors for poor health (11). In a 2005 study (12), hopelessness, pessimism, rumination, anxiety and anger were the five negative manners found most directly linked to cardiovascular disease, while research in 2009 identified neurotic tendencies such as anxiety, worry and depression to increase the risk of mortality in all cases (13). Long-running research has also concluded that pessimistic attitudes were significantly associated with poorer physical and mental functions 30 years later (14).

One particularly interesting experiment directly demonstrates the beneficial effects of consciously bringing one's thoughts in-line with positive ideas. In this study called *Count Blessings versus Burdens* (15), subjects were asked to make regular journal entries for a specific period of time. One group was instructed to record things for which they were grateful (i.e., they were "counting their blessing"), while another was instructed to record things they found annoying and/or irritating. The results revealed not only a much greater sense of overall well-being for the "grateful" group, but also social and physical benefits for them.

I believe that deep down inside we, to some degree or another, know that this power exists within us. Yet in modern times we have been conditioned so firmly to doubt anything that science has not yet presented overwhelming empirical evidence for, that we end up, unknowingly, through our own subconscious doubts and fears, causing the very diseases and medical problems that we inherently have the power to avoid.

Chapter 5:

≈ The Thought Bug ≈

The Thought Bug

Our thoughts don't just affect us personally. They affect our external environment too. Just as all those thought undulations react upon their respective levels *(koshas)* of the individual, these mental vibrations also radiate out from each of us in all directions, affecting the mental bodies *(manomaya koshas)* of others around us too. In other words, thought is infectious.

Thought Emissions

The degree to which a thought can radiate, and as a result affect the mental bodies of others, is directly proportional to both the distance from its source and its level of intensity. This is pretty similar to how the strength and clarity of someone's voice determines the distance that it can penetrate in waves of sound radiating through the air from the speaker to the ears of the listener. In this same way, a strong thought will carry much farther than a weak one, and a clear, decisive thought will take hold more firmly than an uncertain or an ambiguous one.

However, the degree to which a *potentially infectious* thought vibration can affect another person also depends upon the degree of receptivity of the person receiving it. Just as a voice may "fall upon the deaf ears" of someone whose attention is focused upon other things, a thought can easily pass by unnoticed by another whose mind is absorbed in other thoughts. But most people's whole attention is rarely engaged, and so the majority of minds are predominantly in a state where they can, to some degree or another, be affected by (or are receptive to) the thoughts of others that encroach upon them.

What about people whose minds seem to be filled with relentless chatter and activity? This seems like a bit of a paradox because it would suggest that these folks aren't easily affected by the thoughts of others, yet they also seem to be the ones who are usually being shaped the most by the human activities and commotion in their midst. In contrast, someone else might have a calm demeanor and a relatively tranquil mind, but seem to deflect persistent mental assaults of a disruptive nature with ease. How is that?

To resolve this apparent discrepancy, there is a significant qualification to add to the previous assertion. When it comes to being either *receptive* or *closed-off* to external thought waves, what is most important is not the amount of activity already going on within the receiver's mind, but rather their ability to focus their attention and to concentrate on whatever it is that their mind is occupied with.

It is this "hold" of one's mind that inhibits other things (thoughts) from entering, not merely the amount of stuff going on in their head, so to speak. Hence, someone who has discipline and relatively strong mental control is able to quiet (or focus) their mind and remain better insulated from external thought influences. Someone who can sit in meditation on the corner of a busy downtown intersection during rush hour and remain as unaffected as they would be sitting under a tree in the park is demonstrating that. The person who has gained the ability to control the activities of their mind and maintain it in a state of serenity and relative emptiness (or rather, freedom from superficial chitter-chatter) can exit in any bustling environment without damaging effects.

We can also be very focused in an obsessive way, which doesn't necessarily suggest a conscious ability to control the mind. The classic road rage is a perfect example of this. The mind becomes so consumed with a thought – locked into it, you can say that it also precludes them from being affected by the thoughts of others around them. Notice what happens in a situation such as this? How this kind of intensity of thought quickly boils up into the *pranamaya kosha* (emotional body) creating such an extreme state that all thought and ability to reason becomes temporarily suspended. We've probably all witnessed someone who was in such a fury that there was literally "no talking any sense into them." Maybe that person was you?

To a further degree, the person who is *mentally scattered* and whose mind is just a market place of transient, disjointed and fragmented thoughts will be the biggest of receptacle for thought undulations in their external environment. They will find cities and crowded, congested places terribly difficult and uncomfortable surroundings to be in.

How Thoughts From Others Affect Us

If you are sympathetic, that is to say, of the mind that will easily accept a radiating thought from another person, then the effect upon you could be an exact replication of the thought emanating from the other person who produced it.

This is probably not going to happen. It's more likely that the external thought being absorbed by you would produce an effect along lines broadly similar to it. For example, if your friend has a strong feeling of hunger, perhaps a craving for a big fat steak, then when those thought vibrations strike upon the emotional or mental body of another meat-eater, they may arouse in him or her that same type of craving. However, if you're a vegetarian, and your friend's thought vibrations radiate to you, though they might still arouse feelings of hunger, you'll likely have cravings for vegetarian food instead. So, though it is not possible to affect others with a thought that is wholly unfamiliar to them, it (the thought) will influence all those people around it in various ways, according to their present mental state and their own predispositions. On the flip side, someone might also be in a less-sympathetic state, or be less receptive to a particular thought vibration for various reasons. Using the example above, for instance, someone may have just finished a large meal and their appetite has been fully satisfied when they encountered this mental wave of hunger from another. Though they may not have a strong immediate urge to eat another meal because of it, there could be a tendency to engage, to some degree or another, in the act of eating – like having some tea, or squeezing in a little snack or a dessert. Have you ever arrived at a function or party of some sort with an already full belly, but found yourself nibbling away amongst a ravenous crowd in front of a scrumptious spread of food?

The Thought Virus

General *psychic infection* is a well-documented phenomenon throughout history. It can occur within the whole spectrum of mental activity, from pure, kind and uplifting thoughts, to evil, depressive and hate filled thoughts – and everything in between. We see manifestations of this every day, most palpably in group situations – for example, a religious gathering which creates an atmosphere of the highest, joy-filled feelings; or in the opposite instance, the angry mob-mentality of a crowd of protesters hell-bent on mayhem and destruction.

Even on a much smaller scale, by taking careful notice, we see the workings of this principle of thought resonance in the interpersonal interactions we have with those that we come into contact with on a daily basis, unintentionally showering others with the clutter of mental activity going on within us. I've noticed with myself in an annoyed frame of mind spreading the same agitation to someone else who was otherwise quite cheerful until they had the unfortunate opportunity to cross my path at that very moment when I just needed to vent! On the other hand, I've also been aware of a deep sense of peace and tranquility within me specific times, and used that unshakable state of mind to diffuse the stress of someone else that was on a downward spiral of their own.

As you can begin to see, we have a great responsibility for our own thoughts, while the necessity for paying close attention to how the thoughts of others maybe affecting us is also very apparent. Just as unintentionally we are affecting those around us with our negative attitudes and obsessions, we are also, unknowingly, being affected by negative mental influences from others in our midst. The great news is that we also have the potential to do just the opposite, and spill joy, serenity and peace in our wake, without discrimination for the betterment of all who are fortunate enough to pass our way. With that in mind, it makes sense that by positioning ourselves among those who radiate "higher" thoughts, we stand to benefit from the fallout of their elevated spirits, and vice versa. That's why all spiritual traditions, Yoga included, stress the importance of bonding with a like-minded, spiritually ambitious community when embarking on the evolutionary journey.

Like Attracts Like

You know the classic "love at first site" – two people who have happened into contact with each other at the precise moment when both of their minds were already attuned to a similar wave. How about when someone said something, that just moments before, you already knew that they were going to say. Another time you uttered the exact same words in synchronicity with another person for no apparent reason – or you heard someone say exactly what you were thinking at the very moment.

Those are all examples of attuning to the resonance of the thoughts of others around us. It happens without knowledge, without intention, and after a moment or two of bewilderment, we usually just forget all about it. Well, maybe not the love at first site.

But what if we could actually gain some control of it – this power to influence others with our thoughts? Can we deliberately or even unknowingly direct that influence of our thought power? The answer is yes, we can – and people do it all the time.

A Potent Device

In the same way that our thoughts can radiate into our surrounding environment in a *diffuse* manner, our *specific intention* can lend a more exactness to those mental waves. In a way, this could be looked at as a thought that has great intensity (strength, clarity and focus), as I suggested earlier, increases the potential of that thought to affect another person. When that strength, clarity and focus is directed toward a specific person or thing, it delivers itself thereto with marked precision. At the same time it might still affect others in the surrounding area in a more understated manner.

This can be illustrated by the example of someone directing a thought toward someone else, such as feelings of love, hate, anger, jealousy, admiration, etc. Though most everyone within the sphere of the radiating waves created by this thought will be affected by them in some low key way, the *definite intention* attached to the thought directs its primary power straight to the person it is concerned with. How does this thought affect that person? The same conditions apply as mentioned earlier for the radiating thought waves that affect everyone in their path – meaning that the specific person, or recipient, must also be receptive to the thought. If their mind is passive, or has within it oscillations of a nature similar to the incoming thought, then their mind will be immediately and perhaps even strongly affected by it. But if the mind of the recipient is sufficiently occupied by other things, then this thought can penetrate only in so far as the recipient's mind has left room for it to enter.

Let's Get it Together

I frequently notice two people engaged in conversation in a café or a social gathering, where it's all too often apparent that neither one of them is really interested in what the other is saying. Sometimes it seems to be a peculiar game of verbal tennis, where one person is so preoccupied with their own thoughts that they appear only to be merely waiting for the other to stop speaking so that they can continue illustrating their own point of view. All the while they put forth little attention and effort toward ingesting and understanding what their "playing partner" is saying.

That's a good example of the state of the typical person's mind today, which is why, individually, most people's thought-power is actually quite weak, or indecisive. That is to say, their ability to affect others and their surrounding environment is rather insignificant. So unless a person is in a highly charged, focused frame of mind, like the road rage example earlier, they are unlikely to greatly affect, as a solitary individual, others within their immediate environment.

This changes; however, with the strength of a collective effort. Within a bustling market place, for instance, the mind of the average, undisciplined person eventually becomes overwhelmed. The collective jumbled mental activities of hundreds of unrefined minds combine to wreak havoc on all who stray unwittingly into its web.

This illustrates the point that, where individually, a mind may have little strength, collectively they can become a colossal force. So groups of people working together with intentional thought can and will have a much more powerful effect, even extending over much greater distances to their intended object. We see examples of this in group sessions for healing, meditation, etc., which endeavor to do just that. The idea is that, collectively, thoughts can be sent over great distances to facilitate healing in someone who is sick, or to aid others in need in various other ways.

Our united efforts can and do have effects on almost every aspect of life around the globe today, from influencing nature, to the political and social environments. With directed and intentional constructive thoughts and attitudes, humanity possesses a potent resource for positively influencing its own destiny as well as the destiny of the entire planet.

I Think – That's What I Am!

More commonly today we see examples of specific thoughts being directed toward one's self in the form of self criticism, self doubt, self loathing, and self deprecation; perhaps the opposite too, of self glorifying, self adoring notions. In either case, the mechanism is the same. In a similar way to how our thought waves affect others, as long as our own mind is temporarily occupied with business or other concentrated thought, we might remain unaffected by our own negative thought tendencies. But, over time, the constant repetition of negative thoughts can eventually establish a pattern so strong, that as soon as our mind has relaxed its external concentration, it immediately resumes this stream of self-indulgence. This is the underlying force behind neurotic tendencies such as worry, anxiety, and even depression.

Many people who fall victim to this modern tendency find themselves eventually trapped in a self-perpetuating cycle of personally damaging mental activity, where the only relief comes in actively seeking mental distraction, such as immersing oneself in a work environment, television or video games, becoming absorbed in mental fantasies, or grasping onto other mental diversions. This state of mind is extremely limiting to the evolution of the Higher Self, and is perhaps one of the most devastating pathologies that can befall someone. If this tendency is not combated with affirmative action, it can do a great deal of harm over both the short and long-term, ultimately completely suffocating one's ability to evolve.

The Power for Physical Manifestation

Thought has the power to affect physical matter in the external, material world, as certain as it displays the power to influence our inner environment. To understand how this is possible we need to look at what the Yogis consider the fundamentals of [manifest] existence.

Cosmic Vibrations

As stated earlier, physicists have now substantiated that everything in the manifest world is essentially reducible to states of vibration. Similarly, whilst in states of deep resonance with Cosmos (i.e., while in mediation), the Rishis, the ancient yoga scientists perceived that everything manifest, as well as un-manifest, exists within its own frequency, or vibration. What evolved out of their discoveries was the ancient language known as Sanskrit, which is a "verbal approximation" of these *bijas*, or "root universal vibrations." The Rishis discovered that everything in nature possesses its own unique sound, or "sound name," a sort of sound recipe comprised of these elemental sounds *(bijas)* of the Universe. In fact, perfect pronunciation of Sanskrit words, they explained, can replicate the exact vibratory nature of that which it is referring to. Hence, within in the Sanskrit language, everything in the world had been named, not by whimsical notions, fancies or limited perceptions, but as a direct observation of the "Cosmic sound" or vibration that is its essence. It is told then, that if one's mind was utterly pure, then upon hearing this perfectly pronounced symbol (Sanskrit word), the image of that object, idea, etc.., would immediately appear within the mind and the "field of understanding" of this individual, even if they had never seen or heard of it before.

Likewise, the perfect pronunciation of a Sanskrit word (i.e., the perfect enunciation of the vibration associated with a given object or force) has the power to manifest and/or influence that particular thing. Sanskrit, for the very reason that it is the closet verbal approximation of the vibrational spectrum of the Cosmos, is referred to as the "perfect language." This is, at heart, the essence of one of the principles behind _mantra_ chanting in the _Vedic_ tradition of ancient India. Today; however, it is doubtful that there are many, if any who possess this precise knowledge and ability of enunciation, nor any pure enough of mind to be able to receive the innate truths of this language upon hearing it. But even though its understanding and use has been watered down and mostly lost through improper and careless use, nonetheless, Sanskrit remains a powerful force to be rediscovered in Yoga.

Thought, by operating on the same underlying Universal principles of resonance as Sanskrit, possesses this equivalent power of manifestation and control in the seen and unseen worlds. One can even direct and control _prana_ (the Universal Life Force) with the mind, which is the principle aim of the aspect of yoga known as _pranayama_. Though not many today can master the use of thought either at this highly refined or subtle level, it, like the verbal Sanskrit, remains a powerful force to be rediscovered – a force with which one can potentially affect the elements, disturb physical matter, and create and influence everything within the whole spectrum of the existence.

Chapter 6:

≈ The Evolution of the Mind ≈

The Evolution of the Mind

Given the aforementioned yoga understanding of the nature of thought, we could easily conclude that the issue of "thought" is not only of great importance to our (spiritual) evolution, but also in our day to day life, not to mention as a consequence for society as a whole, as well. Since every thought (vibration) we initiate inevitably reacts upon our self and upon those within our external environment, then a great deal of care must be taken as to what thoughts and emotions we allow our self to have.

Highly "evolved" individuals, existing in a more *sattvic* (refined awareness) state, exhibit this consideration, while the vast majority of individuals today, acting often under the influence of what science terms the unevolved "animal brain," rarely think of attempting to check an emotion, and merely yield to the thoughts and reactions that spring forth as a matter of instinctual or conditioned responses. Most of us probably consider ourselves to be well beyond the influence of such a thing as an animal brain, but this part of our nature still plays a strong roll in our existence and, for better or worse, most of us still operate heavily under its influence.

EVOLUTIONARY QUIRKS
By: Yogacharini Meenakshi Devi Bhavanani

Many problems facing the average individual are not his/her own personal problems at all, but rather difficulties common to each and every member of the human race. In the long evolutionary enfoldment from the first form of life – the virus, 3.5 billion years ago – through the fishes (375 million years ago), the amphibians (345 million), the reptiles (300 million), right up to the mammals (60 million years), the accumulated "conditioned responses" of various life forms to environmental challenges have produced organisms which adapted and lived, or failed to adapt and died. The Highest Truth, the Greatest Success of the reptilian and animal kingdoms, is survival.

Somewhere between 40 thousand and 100 thousand years ago – a relatively recent period in the grand scheme of evolution – a great evolutionary event occurred. A mysterious force penetrated the dull, conditioned stimulus-response, pain-pleasure planes of [the animal] existence – and *manas* (or consciousness) manifested on the earth plane. A new creature, a being with the power to think, to reason beyond its genetic inheritance, rose above animal-reptilian instincts. He or she was called "man" or "human" – literally a being that possesses *"manas."* The force of that powerful evolutionary leap propelled the four-legged animal onto two legs and prompted the growth of a new brain structure – the neo-cortex and the pre-frontal lobes of the brain. Or, was it the other way around? Did the new brain structure develop, enabling the "new being" to manifest consciousness? Which came first, the chicken or the egg?

Whatever the cause-effect sequence, this new creature rose out of the conditioning of millions of years of fish-amphibian-reptilian-mammalian experiences. But, all these ancient instincts are still present in his brain structure. These old instincts and conditioned responses enable his heart to beat automatically and his breath to move in and out of his lungs systematically, 21,600 times per day. These old sections of his brain enable him to digest his food and eliminate it; to seek out a mate and procreate; to nurture his offspring and defend his family; to play and frolic in sheer exuberance of the life force. These old remnants of a past long gone are still present in the new being's "old brain" – the brain stem, the limbic system, the reptilian and mammalian complexes.

Although, it is here that a "snag" has developed, an "evolutionary lag" so to speak. These old structures prompt ancient responses to modern challenges, often totally out of proportion to the current situation. The old mammalian emotions produce adrenalin surges, which stimulate fright-flight responses to life and death challenges and appropriate physiological manifestations – the emptying of bowels and bladder, sweaty palms and feet, rapid breath and heart beats. This physiological change was useful when being pursued by a sabre-tooth tiger but becomes extremely useless and even harmful when it is triggered by the fact that one's colleague at the office has gotten a promotion that one expected for one self, or when someone else snatches a much needed train reservation from right under one's nose by cutting the queue. These relatively mundane threats often prompt life and death responses such as rapid heart beat, and adrenalin rushes with a desire to attack, etc. Usually, due to social conditioning, these autonomic responses are curbed, but sometimes the residues linger sub-consciously, causing undefined anxiety attacks, high blood pressure, circulatory and respiratory disorders and so on.

The old sections of the brain also trigger various other survival mechanisms – a sense of hierarchy in relationship to other creatures, a drive for territorial conquests, a thirst for power, seeking dominance in the herd, jealousy, rage, the killing instinct, desire to "eat or be eaten" by the other. These are all "blind passions," the animal instincts so vital to survival in the jungle, which reign in these old segments of the brain.

In so-called modern civilized man," these "basic animal drives" have become more subtle but they still exist in the fiercely competitive worlds of business, sports, media, religious, organizational power struggles, and of course, politics. The need to prove one self " the best," the "top dog," which is so essential for success in any competitive activity, can be traced right back to the old brain and the organism's developing instinct to be the most fit so that it will win the sexual sweepstakes and ensure that its genes will be passed to the next generation. The only difference between the behavior of humans and animals in these matters is that the drives have become more abstract for humans – more subtle – while various types of social restraints evolved by the culture keep them in check.

The new being, the human who walks upright on the earth, also now possesses consciousness – a beam *Manas* or "Consciousness" can perceive beauty, can wonder at this mysterious world, can create tools and shape its own environment. This new being can be dominant and exploit lower life forms. Consciousness opened a huge window to the universe. Man could now look at the sky and see the stars and the great heavens. He could ponder his own fate and wonder at the mysteries of life and death. He now had the power of abstraction and was freed of the prison of sensory information alone ...

This new being is literally "half animal – half man," a creature struggling toward the light, but chained to the past by the fetters of old primordial instincts and drives. This struggle, mirrored in all great world religions, all great art and all the great human myths, is the struggle of every human to rise out of his primordial past and dwell in his true "God-like" nature.

This inherent human problem, "the beast's attempt to become the beauty," is part of the Great Universal Scheme to unfold the individual soul (the *jiva*), leading it to its ultimate destination – Union with the Universal, the *Paramatma*. This is the great dramatic saga of the transformation of the "(Ego) personality" into the "Universality."

When the animal rises up onto two legs and the skull expands forward – when the pre-frontal lobes develop and consciousness is able to find a suitable instrument through which to manifest, an entirely new element enters into the evolutionary scheme of things. The new creature can utilize this consciousness to accelerate its own evolution into a "higher form of being." It has the potential to no longer be a prisoner of past conditioning. It can break free ... It can now make aware choices in its responses to environmental stimuli and challenges. It is no longer an animal ... It is then that *"yoga"* or the "unitive impulse" may be embraced ... The new creature can now evolve itself consciously ... Ignorance can be destroyed by consciously seeking higher and higher levels of Truth. One must free one self of blind animal passions, and consciously strive toward nobility of living ... Realizing that the sense of "I-ness" is an illusion, that in reality, there is only "Oneness" must transcend ego. When personality fades away, Universality emerges ... The lure of pleasure must be seen for the false mistress that it is and the horror of pain must also be seen as an imposter, unworthy of fear ... Finally, one must root out the animal desire to survive at all costs by realizing that one is not the body, but in actuality, one's true being is the Universal Spirit which can never die.

Elevating Our Thoughts

If thought ultimately has the power to uplift humanity, then it is obvious that possessing the capability to create and maintain higher thoughts is essential. This capacity; however, is sorely lacking in the majority who inhabit the earth today. Most of the thought of the average person center around himself, his emotions, his desires, etc., and are of a lower form, dwelling in the lower regions of the energy fields (energy bodies). As a result, in the majority of people the lower aspects (the physical and emotional bodies) are the most active, while the higher, more subtle regions remain underdeveloped, even dormant, harboring little activity. For most folks, in fact, the whole of their "mental atmosphere" is surging with vibrations belonging to the lowest subdivisions, with comparatively little activity happening within the high aspects of their being. If the highest potential of thought is to be realized, it's of primary importance for each of us to first develop this capability for "higher" thought. That should, by now, be pretty evident.

This is precisely the point where the necessity for spiritual study is apparent, be it Yoga, or another disciplined approach to the examination, understanding, development and application of "Universal Truths" in one's life. Except for one thing ...

The average person could really care less about that. It's not their fault, mind you. In so many ways we are a product of our environment, and let's face it, the modern world doesn't exactly nurture and promote the highest ideals of humanity all the time. The average person being a product of this fast-paced, highly competitive, increasingly depersonalized world is more often than not a hub of restless vibrations, constantly in a state of worry, depression, excitement or preoccupation, all the while unaware that they are negatively influencing those around them by the condition of their mental and emotional *(pranic)* bodies.

This is why metropolitan environments are very difficult for the sensitive, spiritually ambitious person to live in. The average, insensitive person who lies in such an environment is also constantly absorbing the vibrations of thousands, or even millions of people who are unnecessarily agitated by all sorts of desires, feelings, and foolish thoughts, and in turn, re-emitting these vibrations back out into this same environment, supporting a perpetual increasingly negative atmosphere where one can no longer be wholly responsible for one's own feelings, thoughts, attitudes or actions. It surely would take a high degree of mastery over your "mental self" in order to live in such an environment without endangering your health and stifling your own evolution.

Compounded by the millions of people around the world today who are virtually "locked into" such states of mind, the unified force created is having severely negative repercussions on the collective consciousness, and hence the overall behavior of humanity. One might even surmise that we are actually "devolving" as a species now and doing so at an alarmingly accelerated rate. Turn on the nightly news and you might very well think that could be the case.

I am reminded of the comment from, Dr. Swami Gitananda Giri Gurumaharaj. He said, "There is really only one sin, and that is the sin of standing in the way of another's (right to) evolution." Unwittingly, most all of us on a day-to-day and moment-to-moment basis, through our own ignorance and lack of awareness, and through our uncontrolled and irresponsible thought, are surely committing that offense.

Chapter 7:

≈ Control Your Mind, Control Your Life ≈

What To Do?

Instead of letting our thoughts and emotions run off here and there, we need to gain their control. Though, we need to consider a few things before we do that.

Our current stage of (spiritual) evolution is a primary factor; I know that this can be a sensitive notion for a lot of people. Due to much of the conditioning we've had, especially in Western cultures, this idea that one person may be more evolved (be it spiritually, emotionally, intellectually or whatever) than someone else can automatically provide thoughts of an authoritative hierarchy and a knee-jerk response something to the effect of, "What makes you think you are better than me?"

It's interesting that this type of "taking offence" at the mere idea that some are more spiritually advanced than others does not exit in what we might call more spiritually-based cultures, such as some of those from the East. In fact, the opposite may even be true, where the average person is much more aware and humbly frank about their own spiritual shortcomings, and have reverence for those that have demonstrated a greater understanding of these things and have offered to help others to benefit from their knowledge and experience.

The irony is that in the West we see this humble, reverential nature as weakness, and not strength. In the West, we don't like the idea that someone may know something that we don't, especially if that knowledge is about us! It's an unfortunately deep *samskara* in Western culture, and one that really presets a big hurdle on the evolutionary journey, holding back so many people from realizing their greater potential in life.

Regaining Control of the Ship

In order to gain control over this unruly force of thought the first thing we need to be clear about is that the mind is not the person. Your thoughts are not YOU. Rather, the mind is an instrument, a tool, and like any tool it can be used to do a good job, or to botch things up royally. We must learn to use the mind properly and effectively. It should not be left uncultivated or allowed to remain idle for any passing "thought influence" to impress upon it. As the saying goes, "The Devil finds work for idle hands (minds)." The mind left unguarded will have a definite tendency toward waywardness, so the first step toward control of the mind is keeping it usefully occupied.

Needles to say, we should always strive to keep our thoughts and activities of a positive and beneficial nature. Even when we're physically idle, we should still maintain positive mental activity. The "*bhakti-drenched*" Saints of India (of whom the Bengali Saint, Ananda Mayi Ma, was one of the famous) is where this behavior was exemplified. Whose minds were ceaselessly attached to thoughts of love for, and devotion to the Divine. Yoga *sadhaks,* or aspirants, at all stages along the spiritual path work towards crafting persistent, higher thoughts. Mental *mantras*, cultivated as a backdrop to our daily activities, are powerful tools for maintaining purity and loftiness of mind.

Similarly, the non-yogi can benefit from establishing a mental panorama of positive affirmations – pleasant thoughts of people, faces, memories, or even ideals. By cultivating a positive, optimistic outlook, the non-yogi develops the ability to hold fast to these things in coexistence with other "worldly" mental demands, not to mention even when the mind is simply at leisure.

The Three Essentials: Awareness, Concentration and Willpower

Such an ideal state of mind may seem out of reach for underdeveloped minds. But there is always hope, and change can always happen if one is truly willing. That change isn't always easy though, and it may take several steps and a considerable amount of time to get there. So many traditions speak about the necessity of a spiritually ambitious approach to life, which is the foundation of evolutionary living. There are many degrees to what can be seen as a spiritually ambitious approach to life. It doesn't mean that we have to relinquish all our possessions and join a religious order, although if that suits your temperament, then this may be your path. It doesn't mean that we need to persuade and convert others, or turn into some kind of religious freak, so to speak. If you've understood the logic I've presented so far, then you can see that those things can just as easily be rooted in *samskara* and unhealthy conditioning as any other passions or obsessions in life.

No, to live a spiritually ambitious life does not mean, more than anything, to simply have a continuous urge to strive for something greater than our own self or satisfying our material desires and attachments – things that will ultimately not bring us the joy and peace we truly want. It means simply to have a "higher marker" that we follow, no matter what direction we choose for our life. Within this higher attitude toward life, there are three important characteristics that need to be cultivated in order to maintain control over our thoughts. They are: awareness, concentration and willpower.

Awareness

To begin gaining control over our mental environment, developing awareness is of prime importance. Before we can affect change within ourselves, we have to first be aware of what needs to be changed and perhaps more importantly, why. Cultivating awareness is the start of lifting the veil of illusion that most people on the globe exist under today, and the device for looking behind that veil to perceive the underlying truths of our existence. As my dear Amma often reminds her students, the first thing that one must become aware of is how unaware they actually are! Most people may assume that because they are cognizant of some of the movements and physical activity around them, because they can carry on a conversation, because they receive good grades in school, because they can dress themselves, hold down a job and otherwise function on a day to day basis without dying, that they must be in possession of the faculty of awareness. Yes, that's true, they are – but the awareness to function at this level is really just a "gross consciousness." It would be quite a stretch of the term awareness, according to the yogis. The awareness that they speak of goes much further than that.

One of the primary functions of many of the practices of yoga is the cultivation of a more "subtle" awareness, which we need in order to be able to perceive what is really going on in our minds – where all our thoughts are actually originating. In order to adjust our thoughts and our actions and reactions, we must be aware of not only what they are, but "why" they are. So the cultivation of awareness and the development of a more refined degree of perception is the cornerstone of an evolving life.

What differentiates humans from lower forms of life is our ability to become aware of how things work –

not only things in our external world, but also ourselves – what makes us tick, physically, mentally and emotionally, so to speak. This is the first stage of what the yogis would refer to as "evolutionary consciousness." Through the process of *svadyaya*, which is the yogic concept of self-study, or the study of the inner workings of one's own mind, we can begin to uncover the conditioned patterns of thought and behavior, attachments, desires, delusions and denials that we may be living under without being fully aware of them. This really is the spiritual path, and so it can be well argued that, unless we are willing to take an honest and frank look at ourselves, and willing to explore life from a deeper and more meaningful perspective, then our ability to achieve any "real awareness" will be quite limited. Only through greater awareness can we begin to recognize the negative activity within our mind and the real problems it is causing us. With that awareness, we can then take a much more proactive stance toward better health and wellbeing.

Concentration

The power of concentration is important in pretty much everything we do, if we want to do it well. No artist ever created a masterpiece while he or she was distracted all the time. No scientific discovery was ever made over beers and casual chit-chat. Deep spiritual insight does not arrive on the scene without the ability to peer deeply into the unknown with focus and great attention.

Developing better concentration ability takes effort – a fair bit more than just, say, trying to "concentrate more," or trying to "pay more attention." Modern minds are jam-packed with *chitta vritti* (mental chatter), preoccupations, obsessions, worries and distractions. In yoga, there are many such structured practices for improving and honing concentration. It's important to note; however, that concentration and meditation is not the same thing, at least not from the yogic perspective. What most people term today as "meditation" is actually, in practice, merely one method or another for developing concentration, or *dharana* as it is called in Yoga. *Dharana* is only a precursor and prerequisite to the higher mental state of meditation, or *dhyana* in Yoga.

With this in mind, the vast majority of popular "meditation techniques" being taught today are perhaps more accurately called practices for helping to develop concentration. Although, the actual value of many of these practices is up for debate, some of them are nonetheless very useful for developing the ability to concentrate better and hence, in helping one to gain mastery over their mental activity – even though they may not yet be adequately prepared for or capable of attaining the higher state of *dhyana*. To really develop strength of concentration though, a consistent and disciplined effort is usually necessary. In the yogic approach, there is a systematic approach to achieving this ability, which involves practices such as focusing attention on the breath or on visual focal points, reciting mental *mantras (ajapa japa),* or various rhythmic breathing exercises and visualizations, to name a few.

It goes without saying that a fair amount of effort is also necessary to strengthen our power of concentration. It requires more than just making some casual attempts at some concentration techniques, from time to time, or an "on again, off again" routine of practice. Sustained and disciplined practice is important for success, and to be able to do that requires a certain amount of willpower – our third consideration.

Willpower

Strength of will, in general, seems to be decreasing in the world today just as humanity on most every technological and scientific front seems to be making positive strides by leaps and bounds. But as our societies are becoming more complex and more demanding at an ever-accelerating rate, people the world over are suffering from an ever-increasing inability to perform up to perceived standards.

The pervading ambition of science is to counter this by "conquering the need for effort" in life, relentlessly pursuing new ways to make life easier and to make every conceivable task of daily life as effortless as possible. In doing so, we have unwittingly and ironically rendered ourselves weaker in our ability to make a willful effort if and when the need arises. Willpower, you see, is like a muscle. It is a "mental muscle," and like the physical musculature of the body, if we do not exercise it regularly it will become weak. If we do not use it much at all, then it can deteriorate almost completely.

The majority of tasks of daily living today can be performed within reach of the touch of a button, and down to earth, good old-fashioned physical effort has been replaced with a high-tech, convenient modern lifestyle. As a result, when faced with the burden of effort, that is to say when faced with actually having to do something challenging and requiring uncommon effort both physically and/or mentally, many are unable to see it through to an efficient and effective end. We have become weakened by affluence to the point where the lack of willpower is now endemic.

The ancient yogis may perhaps not have foreseen this degree of degradation in modern society, but they were fully aware of the innate tendency of humans to seek the pleasurable over the difficult and, most often, the easiest course of action in any given circumstance. They were also cognizant of the effects that this behavior has on people's strength of will and consequently its detriment to the evolution of humanity as a whole. Therefore, the yogis have recognized a necessity. They say, "If life is too easy, we should, we must make it harder – for our own good."

Here, the yogic concept of *tapasya* can be a useful means for building up this strength of will. *Tapasya* is often defined simply as "austerity." It comes from the root word *tejas*, meaning, "fire" or "heating up." In the literal sense, it means to "purify through heating." In *Yoga sadhana*, or Yoga practice, it implies intentionally choosing to do something difficult that requires great effort and concentration. By choosing a *tapasya*, or simply a task, a job, or a mission, be it a singular effort or a change to our lifestyle or habits, with the commitment to see it through to its intended end, we develop our strength or will.

By starting with small, challenging, yet manageable tasks, and by gradually increasing the degree of this challenge in successive pledges as each are achieved, we systematically build up our inner resolve. For instance, I might begin with a few "minor" lifestyle changes, such as getting up at an earlier hour in the morning, and also perhaps forgoing sweet desserts after dinner – and then see those efforts through to the point where they become no longer difficult. Then I might move up to adding a more challenging regiment of physical exercise when I get up in the morning, with the determination to also sit silently for a short period each day and perhaps also to reduce the intake of coffee from two to one cup per day. Carrying on like this, I not only begin to re-organize my life into a more healthy way, but I gradually gain control over the habitual pattern of succumbing to each and every passing desire I have, gaining control over them step by step, one by one, and strengthening my ability to overcome other negative tendencies and influences as they present themselves.

In this way, a chronic smoker will be able to eventually build up the ability to kick the habit, where otherwise simply waking up one day with the ambition to quit smoking, without first developing the strength of will, is commonly bound for failure.

Developing the Essentials

There are many aspects concerning the development of awareness, concentration and willpower. For instance, a fundamental principle in nature is that we must already possess (at least a certain amount of) something in order to acquire more of that thing. As the saying goes, "you have to have money to make money." So, when we already have a certain level of awareness, concentration and willpower, then we're in a much better position to develop more of each of these things. As a result, we become much more capable of applying the strengths of these three, in unison, the tasks of our daily life, in purposeful efforts to strengthen each of them even further.

It is true that some degree or another of change is possible for anyone, even for those who might not have a particularly well-developed sense of awareness, concentration capacity or strength of will. A lot of us might be a bit more deficient than we think in any or all of these areas, so making positive strides in developing these talents can take a fair amount of work in the beginning. Like I said, having some of these things to start with makes the task much easier. Unfortunately, though we can borrow money from another to embark on a business venture, we can't simply borrow awareness, concentration or willpower to get us started in this undertaking.

The good news is the fact that we must first possess a small amount of something to be able to get more of it suggests that we all must already, somewhere, have some bit of all of these virtues within us, because we are all certainly capable of developing them further.

Karma has placed us all within our current life situations and skillfully laid out in front of each of us the challenges that are our individual tasks to overcome in this life. But, although obstacles may sometimes seem severe, *karma* never gives us more than we are capable of handling. Finding the resolve and the effort within that is necessary to overcome any and all of the seemingly unfair or disparaging hurdles in our life, is the *dharma* (correct action, according to one's *karma*) of all of us and, if performed sufficiently, will bear fruits.

So there is, somewhere inside all of us, at least some sparks of each of these characteristics of awareness, concentration and willpower, even if it might appear on the surface that there is very little. If those abilities seem weak, the job is to awaken these innate facilities lying dormant within and to develop each of them to a capacity that will drive us onward to higher stages of evolution.

Most of us have never put forth such a conscious effort to develop things like awareness before, so it's usually best to begin at the base level, placing primary attention into the usual, moment-to-moment activities of daily life. Whatever the task at hand, whether it be reading, cooking, driving, or just listening to someone speak, a simple, mindful effort to pay attention should be made. Turn off the television and radio, and eliminate any obvious distractions and just "do" what it is that "you are doing," and nothing else. By continuing to make this small change in the way we do things, slowly and steadily we'll create a greater awareness and develop the ability to concentrate and to gain willful control of our own minds.

We can expand the principle mentioned above, the one about needing to have something in order to gain more of it, to include that the more you gain of something, the easier it gets to acquire even more of it. This explains why our efforts usually outweigh our gains in the beginning. This ratio of efforts to gains decreases exponentially, though, as we successfully make further and further gains – to the point when a higher level of mastery is attained and where gains are revealed in greater proportion to the effort we put forth.

The Double-Edged Sword

The development of thought power can also be a double-edged sword, in that gaining mastery over this potent force is not dependent on a morality, wisdom, or discernment. Anyone who puts their mind to the task with great determination can, to some degree or another, develop a very strong capacity to affect those around them and to manifest anything that they so choose, be it good or bad, beneficial or useless, helpful or harmful.

Of course, many are already unconsciously able to do this as demonstrated by those who have become submerged within a sea of self-deprecation, continually creating for themselves a life of frustrations, disturbances, disappointments, disease, and an overall lack of fulfillment. Similarly, those fueled by an ego-driven, intensely focused, single-minded drive to achieve some goal, be it political, social, material or economic, can and often do exhibit a powerful ability to clear themselves a path to these ends.

Conversely, the great sages and saints of history have demonstrated that with a properly directed effort of similar intensity, one is capable of reaching the highest stages of eternal fulfillment, gaining profound wisdom, boundless joy, lasting peace, and ultimately self-realization.

Cultivating a Fertile Field

As an objective observer, even a passing glance at society reveals that, for the majority much of this "internal environment" lays for the most part undiscovered and/or underdeveloped. In observing the typical behaviors of the average person, it's pretty apparent that a lot of minds are conditioned with many negative tendencies that need rewiring, so to speak. For instance, a lot of folks waste a great deal of energy in needless disagreements. It even appears impossible for many to simply hold any opinion at all – religious, political, or even relating to some ordinary matter in day to day life – without feeling the need to force that opinion upon everyone else. They even seem incapable of grasping the simple fact that what someone else chooses to believe is not business of theirs at all, and that it is not their sole responsibility in this world to go around and secure uniformity in thought and ideas. The sensible person, though, knows that "truth" has many dimensions, and is not the sole possession of one particular individual of group. He/she also knows that most of the topics over which people consume their energy in opposition are hardly even worth the trouble of discussion, and that those who speak the loudest and the most often are usually the ones who really know the least.

The wise do not get caught in the "trap of logic" either, because they know that this tool of the mind is not a sound barometer of truth, and that someone who has mastered the craft of "logical argument" can easily turn the most absurd of untruths into a favorable light.

The wise person; however, is quite willing to give their opinions and share what they know if asked, but declines to waste time in foolish argument and unprofitable squabbling. He/she not only accepts that others may have different views, but eagerly

86

listens to them, considering that there may be opportunity to expand their own understanding and perspective by doing so.

Let's All Take a Chill Pill

Another, and perhaps the most common waste of energy, is worry. We only need to take a short survey of those around us to be astounded by the spectrum of ridiculous things that people have gotten themselves "tied up in knots of worry" about. It truly can be mind-boggling. Certainly, modern society has thrust upon the shoulders of its unsuspecting members, a vast array of common troubles to fret, agonize and lose sleep over. Financial fears, security for themself and loved ones, the fear of dying or of impending traumas or calamities all have created a commonly high stress level that pervades our space today. Many people are so consumed by these negative vibrations within their emotional bodies that almost every concern that arises throughout the course of normal daily life also becomes a cause for foolish worry – "the bus is five minutes late ... Oh my GOD ... AHHHHHH!"

But again, the wise person knows that just laws govern the Universe, and although we may run, we cannot hide from that which is due to us. The insightful person knows that whatever comes their way is necessary for their own evolution, and that needlessly worrying about things that are out of our control only takes away valuable time and energy that could be better spent cultivating greater understanding to help us to advance further along the compulsory path – one that we all must tread, back to the Divine. Knowing that worry never helps, nor has it ever been of even the slightest use, the intelligent person goes about their business the best that they can, assured that all will be well for them. It is within this understanding that a prudent person is able to free him/herself from worry and cultivate a state of *stitha prajna* (equanimity), peace, contentment and joy in all circumstances.

If we are wise, we refuse to engage in confrontation, or to allow our self to react with negative emotion as a result of the actions of others, realizing that nothing anyone can say or do can cause us emotional distress. If we feel distressed in any way, it is purely and solely of our own doing, in choosing to react that way. With an evolved state of mind, one remains eternally in control of their emotional state and is able to go about their business without the slightest care or concern for the opinions or foolish, spiteful remarks of others.

But in order to display this higher state of understanding and discernment without waver we need the strength of will, maturity and dignity that results from genuine (and honest) study of our own inner environment (*svadyaya*), coupled with a disciplined effort to re-organize our own conditioned psyche.

Responsibility

It is of the utmost importance that we strive to curb these negative mental tendencies, not only for our own personal evolution, but in order to also contribute a positive influence in a largely negative sea of human mental activity. Each time we fail to curb negative mental activity, we create or re-enforce structures of patterned behaviors and responses (*samskaras*) within our mind, which will lend more weight toward prompting that same response again and again in similar circumstances. In short, we create bad unconscious mental habits that make resisting negative inputs even more difficult the next time that they arrive.

Every time we fail to curb a negative mental reaction, we also arouse similar vibrations in the mind or the energy body of those within our sphere of influence – creating these thoughts if they are not present in another already, or intensifying them if they were previously there, This making the evolutionary work of our fellow human beings a little bit more difficult.

The responsibility that each of us has is, therefore, quite apparent. As suggested previously, we need to first become aware, and then become capable of controlling our mental activity, or else unknowingly, like spreading infectious germs, we'll continue to cause undue harm to others and play our own, not-so-insignificant role in the further degradation of humanity. Conversely, if we radiate calmness, equal mindedness, love, compassion, understanding, wisdom and other virtuous mental vibrations, then we achieve exactly the opposite – becoming a distinctly positive influence on those around us who are engaged in the same universal struggle for health and happiness that we are.

Thought is a truly magnificent power, yet its potential is equal in every human being, from the poorest to the wealthiest, from the child to the most learned.

Possessing this tremendous power, we must be careful how we exercise it. What we think about our self will manifest in some way. The thoughts that we harbor of another person will also act powerfully upon them with a force that will tend to pull them toward its fulfillment too. So as we endeavor to concentrate on good thoughts, those that focus on our own positive qualities, as well as those of our friends, we will tend to create new vibrations, or to strengthen those undulations that are already present.

We must be ever diligent and resist the urge to judge or condemn others or to allow ourselves to be drawn into engaging in gossip, rumors or speculations, whether true or untrue, about another person. This is perhaps the most iniquitous and offensive activity that we can allow our self to engage in, yet today it is commonplace behavior, even often for the most pious seeming individuals. This filthy act has become a despicable habit passed down from parents to children and from teachers to students, re-enforced in the media and entertainment industries, and nurtured within a society consumed with the mindless chitter-chatter of modern day life. When rumor surfaces about an individual, even though it may be a baseless one, the collective negative (thought) energy that accumulates when hundreds, or even thousands of people turn their attention toward it can drive that person (the subject of the rumor) into social, political, economic and even mental ruin. We see countless examples of this every day, right in front of us, with the fires of destruction begin fueled by an often-indiscriminate mass media machine, and the political engines behind them.

This is a striking example of how, on a smaller scale such as in our personal lives, we can, and often do inflict unintentional harm upon those who, in many circumstances, are undeserving of any punishment – those who, like ourselves, are not perfect and do sometimes make mistakes, but who could also be much better served by our uplifting thoughts rather than our chastising ones as they struggle along that same path which we are all treading on toward greater understanding, fulfillment and happiness in life. When we gossip and pass our negative notions about someone onto another person, who in turn, may pass it onto another who passes it onto another, and so on and so on, then we have created an exponentially expanding web of people who are, together, directing convergent streams of negative thought toward a certain individual. Together, through the resonance of these collective thoughts, we all aid in creating those very negativities in that person that we gossiped about, which may or may not have been already present in that poor individual to begin with. But even if these negative traits were already present in them, then we end up causing them an additional hurdle in overcoming that weakness, one, which they are probably already struggling to defeat, unsympathetically causing them more unnecessary harm in the end.

Hence, if we know of certain faults or shortcomings in a person, we should avoid letting our thoughts dwell upon them, lest we unwittingly help to strengthen these non-virtuous characteristics of theirs. On the contrary, we do a great service to them by formulating strong thoughts of the opposite nature and sending our waves of those virtuous thoughts to this person who could use our help.

We can still remain genuine in our perception of the imperfections of the others around us, but it's precisely in the way that we choose to react (mentally, verbally, and otherwise) that we need to make moral strides and a positive difference.

As introduced earlier, the yogic concept of *pratipaksha bhavana* literally means, "the opposite point of view." It is the conscious effort to immediately, by an act of will, replace any negative thought, as soon as it arise, with an opposite, more virtuous and positive one – a potent tool not only for our own evolution, but for the betterment of all those around us as well.

Let's think lovingly and warmly of our friends; let's also think lovingly and warmly of those whom we are indifferent to; and let's think lovingly and warmly about our enemies as well. Let's think of their good points and try, by concentrating our attention upon those good points, to strengthen and to help them to become better people as well. Let us celebrate with joy the pearls that lie within each and every person; however, buried or hidden they may seem at the time and let's do this with as much eagerness as the average person whose criticisms are swift to pounce upon an imaginary flaw!

The Rewards of Effort

When attempting to control our thoughts and passions, we'll no doubt fail time and time again and maybe conclude that such an achievement is not possible and that such an effort is useless. Certainly to be successful in the task requires more than just a mere matter of wishing for it. It requires all that I have discussed up until this point, and even more. It's true that some face greater challenges and difficulties than others, but this is not merely the unfortunate circumstances of a randomly dealt hand, as it were. The law of *karma* continually places before us the fruits of our past labors as well as the thorns of our historical negligence. "For whatsoever a man soweth, that shall be also reap" (Galatians 6:7) is a Universal Truth. It doesn't matter whether or not someone has knowledge or memory of what also extends backwards into times of previous lives, as the yogis believe, where they might have unknowingly allowed certain harmful or unfavorable attitudes and characteristics to lay roots within their own mental structure, or whether or not they have unknowingly caused these things to happen throughout this life. Whatever the case may be, we are all different by virtue of our own, unique past, which makes setting ourselves upon a better mental course, a different level of challenge for each of us when we finally do develop the conscious awareness and inclination to do so.

Without a conscious effort to counter these accumulated negative tendencies (*samskaras*), we'd be certain to go on sliding down the same slope, continuing to strengthen and re-enforce our destructive affinities, making the job of overcoming them, a job which we all MUST eventually take on, more and more difficult. But though it's difficult, it's not impossible to overcome this challenge. The amount of energy accumulated – i.e., that energy that supports the maintenance of these *samskaras* within the subtle bodies – is essentially a fixed amount. Even if we have allowed it to build up over several lifetimes, still the accumulated sum is limited. Once we have realized the mistakes we've made and set ourselves out to control those bad habits and counter the impetus, we find that we ultimately only need to put forth as much strength in the opposite direction as we did in setting up the destructive mental tendencies in the first place. Ok, I know that still might seem like a lot of effort, but as the saying goes, "Rome wasn't built in a day."

All of the deeply rooted conditionings in our subconscious didn't appear there overnight either. They were created, built up slowly, over time, and they will be dismantled and replaced the same way. Some subconscious tendencies are definitely going to be deeply rooted, so some time and extra effort will be required to overcome them. We can all take refuge, though, in knowing that effort well spent will eventually yield rewards. Someone who has spent three or four decades abusing their physical body in every conceivable manner, through drugs, alcohol, poor diet, misuse, etc., can't expect to regain perfect health from a month's worth of exercise at the gym. This is equally true with the mental abuses of the past. With determined and persistent effort, though, eventually this "mental neglect" can be mended. Every bit of effort that we make to the contrary will lesson the amount of negative force that has been stored up in our being. As long as we are living, each and every action, thought and word that we commit will have either a positive or negative implication within our mental structure. Therefore, success is purely a matter of choice – or whether we choose to re-enforce old patterns of thought, attitude and behavior through negligence, disinterest and laziness; or whether we choose to break down the damaging mental and emotional structures that hinder our quest for fulfillment and happiness, by creating new, beneficial mental inclinations and mindfully cultivating awareness, universal understanding, truth, compassion and loving attitudes and thoughts.

Let's Make the World a Better Place

One of the greatest powers that we all possess is our ability to use our thought to give assistance to someone who is suffering – and most everyone today is suffering on one level or another. Even though we may not be able to help somebody physically, or though their physical brain may be closed off to our suggestion by prejudice or narrow-mindedness, their mental and energy bodies remain more easily impressionable and are always open to some degree to a wave of helpful thought of caring and calmness. Our steady and concentrated, loving thoughts will eventually find a crack to creep in through. I read the following quote in an old book, which demonstrates just the right mindset:

> "Knead love into the bread that you bake; wrap strength and courage in the parcel that you tie for the woman with the weary face; hand trust and candor with the coin that you pay to the man with the suspicious eyes."

What better attitude could we possibly have when approaching the activities and associations of our daily life? A wonderful, unexpected by-product also results from this mental exercise. All the while, as we are turning our attention to generating and sending benevolent thoughts to others, we no longer have the time to create negative ones within ourselves. Thus, unconsciously and quite unknowingly, we steadily break down our own negative *samskaric* matrix within and replace those destructive attitudes and tendencies with a whole new anthology of *sattvic*, or uplifting inclinations. Along with a constructive personal life design – one based upon the view that we are all one, all part and parcel of the same Divine universal consciousness – we can reframe the picture of our own self, removing the chronic obstacles or preconceived notions and attitudes that have inhibited our success in so many ways on the playing field of life.

We should, therefore, be ever watchful for an opportunity to exercise this power of thought in a beneficial and positive way. With awareness and alertness, it is quite apparent that occasions to do this are plentiful. Even amid the bustling activity of the people that we come across in so many circumstances of our normal daily lives, we might often see someone who is in an obvious state of mental agitation, sadness, or suffering, and take the opportunity to try to help them through the power of positive thought. Every connection is an opportunity and every person that we meet, even casually, is a person to be helped in some way or another.

All who can think can send out kind and useful thoughts. All can, and should do their part to better the world through helpful thoughts toward others. No such thought has ever failed. We may not always see the result, but it is there nonetheless and we don't know what fruits may blossom from the tiny seeds of compassion, love and harmony that we have sown.

Let's go about distributing our blessings on all, doing good aimlessly everywhere we tread, with the recipients all the while unaware to the gift they have received, in the true yogic sense of sincere, unsigned, selfless service to our fellow human beings. Let's endeavor to all living beacons of constructive energy, sending forth the feeling that, in spite of one's personal sorrows and troubles, the sun still shines above each and every one of us, and there is still much to be thankful for, much that is good and beautiful in this world.

... OM

Studies:

Optimism and Re-hospitalization After Coronary Artery Bypass Graft Surgery

Michael F. Scheier, PhD; Karen A. Matthews, PhD; Jane F. Owens, DrPH; Richard Schulz, PhD; Michael W. Bridges, PhD; George J. Magovern, Sr, MD; Charles S. Carver, PhD

Arch Intern Med. 1999;159:829-835.

Objective: To determine whether optimism predicts lower rates of re-hospitalization after coronary artery bypass graft surgery for the 6 months after surgery.

Methods: A prospective, inception cohort design was used. The sample consisted of all consenting patients (N=309) from a consecutive series of patients scheduled for elective coronary artery bypass graft surgery at a large, metropolitan hospital in Pittsburgh, PA. To be eligible, patients could not be scheduled for any other coincidental surgery (ex: valve replacement) and could not be in the cardiac intensive care unit or experiencing angina at the time of the referral. Participants were predominantly men (69.9%), married (80.3%), and averaged 62.8 years of age. Recruitment occurred between January 1992 and January 1994.

Results: Compared with pessimistic persons, **optimistic** persons were significantly less likely to be re-hospitalized for a broad range of aggregated problems (including postsurgical sternal wound infection, angina, myocardial infarction, and the need to another bypass surgery or percutaneous trans luminal coronary angioplasty) generally indicative of a poor response to the initial surgery (odds ratio=0.50, 95% confidence interval=0.33-0.76;*P*=.001). The effect of optimism was independent of traditional socio-demographic and medical control variables, as well as independent of the effects of self-esteem, depression, and neuroticism. All-cause re-hospitalization also tended to be less frequent for **optimistic** than for pessimistic persons (odds ratio=0.77, 95% confidence interval=0.57-1.05;*P*=.07).

Conclusion: Optimism predicts a lower rate of re-hospitalization after coronary artery bypass graft surgery. Fostering positive expectations may promote better recovery.

Dispositional Optimism and the Risk of Cardiovascular Death – The Zutphen Elderly Study

Erik J. Giltay, PhD, MD; Marjolein H. Kamphuis, MSc; Sandra Kalmijn, PhD, MD; Frans G. Zitman, PhD, MD; Daan Kromhout, PhD, MPH

Arch Intern Med. 2006;166:431-436.

Background: Dispositional **optimism**, defined in terms of life engagement and generalized positive outcome expectancies for one's future, may be related to lower cardiovascular mortality. We aimed to determine whether dispositional **optimism** is a stable trait over time and whether it is independently related to lower cardiovascular mortality in elderly men.

Methods: In a cohort study with a follow-up of 15 years, we included 545 (61.4%) of 887 men, aged 64 to 84 years, who were free of preexisting cardiovascular disease and cancer and who had complete data on cardiovascular risk factors and socio-demographic characteristics. Dispositional **optimism** was assessed using a 4-item questionnaire in 1985, 1990, 1995 and 2000. In Cox proportional hazards models, the first 2 years of observation were excluded.

Results: **Optimism** scores significantly decreased over 15 years, but showed temporal stability (reliability coefficients, 0.72 over 5 years and 0.78 over 15 years; $P < .001$). Optimists in 1985 had a hazard ratio for cardiovascular mortality of 0.45 (top tertile vs lowest tertile; 95% confidence interval, 0.29-0.68), adjusted for classic cardiovascular risk factors.

The risk of cardiovascular death was inversely associated with increased tertiles of dispositional **optimism** ($P < .001$ for trend). Similar results were obtained using 1990 data after additional adjustment for depression (assessed by the Zung Self-rating Depression Scale).

Conclusion: Dispositional **optimism** is a relatively stable trait over 15 years and shows a graded and inverse association with the risk of cardiovascular death.

Counting Blessings versus Burdens: An experimental investigation of gratitude and subjective well-being in daily life.
Emmons, Robert A.; McCullough, Michael E.

Current issue feed: Journal of Personality and Social Psychology, Vol. 84(2), Feb. 2003, 377-389.

The effect of a grateful outlook on psychological and physical well-being was examined. In Studies 1 and 2, participants were randomly assigned to 1 of 3 experimental conditions (hassles, gratitude listing, and either neutral life events or social comparison); they then kept weekly (Study 1) or daily (Study 2) records of their moods, coping behaviors, health behaviors, physical symptoms, and overall life appraisals. In a 3rd study, persons with neuromuscular disease were randomly assigned to either the gratitude condition or to a control condition. The gratitude-outlook groups exhibited heightened well-being across several, though not all, of the outcome measures across the 3 studies, relative to the comparison groups. The effect on positive affect appeared to be the most robust finding. Results suggest that a conscious focus on blessings may have emotional and interpersonal benefits.
- Digital Object Identifier:
- 10.1037/0022-3514.84.2.377

Research on Gratitude

Some of the seminal research on the effects of practicing gratitude on a recurring basis was provided via a series of 3 experiences conducted by Emmons and McCullough. In order to maximize the potential generalizability of the results, the sample participants for the first 2 studies consisted of healthy college students, whereas participants in the third study were adults with various congenital and acquired neuromuscular disorders. Within each study, some participants were instructed to maintain a journal on a weekly basis (for 10 weeks) and others, on a daily basis (for 2 or 3 weeks). The entire sample kept records of both positive and negative affects experienced as well as their coping behaviors, health behaviors, physical symptoms, and overall appraisals of life. Subgroups in each study were directed to focus their journal entries on different things:

- Group A recorded things for which they were grateful (ex. They were "counting their blessings")
- Group B recorded things they found annoying and/or irritating
- Group C recorded things that had a major impact on them

When the data from all 3 studies were compiled and analyzed, 2 overarching trends were readily discernable:

1. Participants in the group monitoring things for which they were grateful evidenced higher levels of well-being than those in either of the 2 comparison groups, but particularly when compared to group B (tabulating things they experienced as annoying or irritating).
2. The positive effects of a grateful outlook for participants in the longer study duration (10 weeks vs. 2 or 3 weeks) included not only overall well-being, but social and physical benefits as well.

REF: Emmons RA, McCullough ME. Counting Blessings versus Burdens: an experimental investigation of gratitude and subjective well-being in daily life. *J Pers Soc Psychol.* 2003;84:377-389

http://ccn.aacnjournals.org/cgi/external_ref?access_num=10.1037%2F0022-3514.84.2.377&link_type-DOI

Positive Psychological Well-Being and Mortality: A Quantitative Review of Prospective Observational Studies

Yoichi Chida, MD, PhD and Andrew Steptoe, DPhil

From the Psychobiology Group, Department of Epidemiology and Public Health, University College London, London, UK. Address correspondence and reprint requests to Yoichi Chida, Psychobiology Group, Department of Epidemiology and Public Health, University College London, 1-19 Torrington Place, London WC1E 6BT, UK. Email: y.chida@ucl.ac.uk

Objective: To review systematically prospective, observational, cohort studies of the association between positive well-being and mortality using meta-analytic methods. Recent years have witnessed increased interest in the relationship between positive psychological well-being and physical health.

Methods: We searched general bibliographic databases: Medline, PsycINFO, Web of Science, and PubMed up to January 2008. Two reviewers independently extract data on study characteristics, quality, and estimates of associations.

Results: There were 35 studies (26 articles) investigating mortality in initially healthy populations and 35 studies (28 articles) of disease populations. The meta-analyses showed that positive psychological well-being was associated with reduced mortality in both the healthy population (combined hazard ratio (HR) = 0.82; 95% Confidence Interval (CI) = 0.76-0.89; $P < .001$) and the disease population (combined HR = 0.98; CI = 0.95-1.00; $P = 0.30$) studies. There were indications of publication bias in this literature, although the fail-safe numbers were 2444 and 1397 for healthy and disease population studies, respectively. Intriguingly, meta-analysis of studies that controlled for negative affect showed that the protective effects of positive psychological well-being were independent of negative affect. Both positive affect (ex. emotional well-being, positive mood, joy, happiness, vigor, energy) and positive trait-like dispositions (ex. live satisfaction, hopefulness, optimism, sense of humor) were associated with reduced mortality in healthy population studies. Positive psychological well-being was significantly associated with reduced cardiovascular mortality in healthy population studies, and with reduced death rates in patients with renal failure and with human immunodeficiency virus-infection.

Conclusion: The current review suggests that positive psychological well-being has a favorable effect on survival in both healthy and diseased populations.

Association of Optimism and Pessimism with Inflammation and Hemostasis in the Multi-Ethnic Study of Atherosclerosis (MESA)

Brita Roy, MD, MPH, MS; Ana V. Diez-Roux, MD, PhD; Teresa Seeman, PhD; Nalini Ranjit, PhD; Steven Shea, MD and Mary Cushman, MD
Published online before print January 25, 2010, 10.1097/PSY.0b013e3181cb981b
PSYCHOSOMATIC MEDICINE 72:134-140 (2010)

Low Pessimism Protects Against Stroke

The Health and Social Support (HeSSup) Prospective Cohort Study

Hermann Nabi, PhD; Markku Koskenvuo, MD, PhD; Archana Singh-Manoux, PhD; Jyrki Korkeila, MD, PhD; Sakari Suominen, MD, PhD; Katariina Korkeila, MD, PhD; Jussi Vahtera, MD, PhD; Mika Kivimäki, PhD

From INSERM U687-IFR69 (H.N., A.S.-M), Villejuif, France; the Department of Public Health (M. Koshenvuo), University of Helsinki, Helsinki, Finland; the Department of Epidemiology and Public Health (A.S.-M., M. Kivimäki), University College London, London, UK; the Department of Psychiatry (J.K.), University of Turku and Harjavalta Hospital, Turku, Finland; the Department of Public Health (S.S., J.V.), University of Turku and Turku University Hospital, Turku, Finland; Municipal Health Care (K.K.), Turku, Finland; and the Finnish Institute of Occupational Health (J.V., M. Kivimäki), Helsinki, Finland.

Correspondence to Hermann Nabi, PhD, INSERM Unité 687, 16 Avenue Paul Vaillant Couturier, 94807 Villejuif Cedex, France. Email Hermann.Nabi@inserm.fr

Background and Purpose: The association between optimism, pessimism and health outcomes has attracted increasing research interest. To date, the association between these psychological variables and risk of stroke remains unclear. We examined the relationship between pessimism and the 7-year incidence of stroke.

Methods: A random sample of 23,216 adults (9480 men, 13,736 women) aged 20 to 54 years completed the pessimism scale in 1998, that is, at study baseline. Fatal and first nonfatal stroke events during a mean follow-up of 7-years were documented by linkage to the national discharge and mortality registers leading to 105 events.

Results: Unadjusted hazard ratio was 0.44 (95% CI, 0.25 to 0.77) for participants in the lowest quartile (a low pessimism level) when compared with those in the highest quartile (a high pessimism level). After serial adjustments for socio-demographic characteristics, cardiovascular bio-behavioral risk factors, depression, general feeling of stressfulness, and ischemic heart disease, the fully adjusted hazard ratio was 0.52 (95% CI, 0.29 to 0.93).

Conclusion: In this population of adult men and women, low level of pessimism had a robust association with reduced incidence of stroke.

(CIRCULATION. 2009;120:656-662)

Optimism, Cynical Hostility, and Incident Coronary Heart Disease and Mortality in the Women's Health Initiative

Hilary A. Tindle, MD, MPH; Yue-Fang Change, PhD; Lewis H. Kuller, MD, DrPH; JoAnn E. Manson, MD, DrPH; Jennifer G. Robinson, MD, MPH; Milagros C. Rosal, PhD; Greg J. Siegle, PhD; Karen A, Matthews, PhD

From the University of Pittsburgh (H.A.T., Y.-F.C., L.H.J., G.J.S., K.A.M.), Pittsburgh, PA; Brigham and Women's Hospital and Harvard Medical School (J.E.M.), Boston, MA; University of Iowa (J.G.R.), Iowa City, IA; and University of Massachusetts (M.C.R.), Worchester, MA.

Correspondence to Hilary A. Tindle, MD, MPH, 230 McKee Place, Suite 600, Pittsburgh, PA 15213. Email: tindleha@upmc.edu
Received January 6, 2009; accepted June 18, 2009.

Background: Trait optimism (positive future expectations) and cynical, hostile attitudes toward others have not been studied together in relation to incident coronary heart disease (CHD) and mortality in postmenopausal women.

Methods and Results: Participants were 97,253 women (89,259 white, 7,994 black) from the Women's Health Initiative who were free of cancer and cardiovascular disease at study entry. The Life Orientation Test-Revised and cynical hostility assessed optimism by the cynicism subscale of the Cook Medley Questionnaire. Cox proportional hazard models produced adjusted hazard ratios (AHRs) for incident CHD (myocardial infarction, angina, percutaneous coronary angioplasty, or coronary artery bypass surgery) and total mortality (CHD, cardiovascular disease, or cancer related) over 8 years. Optimists (top versus bottom quartile ["pessimists"]) had lower age-adjusted rates (per 10,000) of CHD (43 versus 60) and total mortality (46 versus 63). The most cynical, hostile women (top versus bottom quartile) had higher rates of CHD (56 versus 44) and total mortality (46 versus 63). Optimists (versus pessimists) had a lower hazard of CHD (AHR 0.91, 95% CI 0.83 to 0.99), CHD-related mortality (AHR 0.70, 95% CI 0.55 to 0.90), cancer-related mortality (blacks only; AHR 0.56, 95% CI 0.35 to 0.88), and total mortality (AHR 0.86, 95% CI 0.79 to 0.93). Most (versus least) cynical, hostile women had a higher hazard of cancer-related mortality (AHR 1.23, 95% CI 1.09 to 1.40) ad total mortality (AHR 1.16, 95% CI 1.07 to 1.27; this effect was pronounced in blacks). Effects of optimism and cynical hostility were independent.

Conclusion: Optimism and cynical hostility are independently associated with important health outcomes in black and white women. Future research should examine whether interventions designed to change attitudes would lead to altered risks.

Emotional Vitality and Incident Coronary Heart Disease
Benefits of Healthy Psychological Functioning

Laura D. Kubzansky, PhD and Rebecca C. Thurston, PhD

Arch Gen Psychiatry. 2007; 64(12):1393-1401.

Context: The potentially toxic effects of psychopathology and poorly regulated emotion on physical health have long been considered, but less work has addressed whether healthy psychological functioning may also benefit physical health. Emotional vitality – characterized by a sense of energy, positive well-being, and effective emotion regulation – has been hypothesized to reduce risk of heart disease, but no studies have examined this relationship.

Objectives: To examine whether emotional vitality is associated with reduced risk of coronary heart disease (CHD). Secondary aims are to consider whether effects are independent of negative emotion and how they may occur.

Design: A prospective population-based cohort study.

Setting: National Health and Nutrition Examination Survey 1 and follow-up studies (a probability sample of US adults).

Participants: 6,025 men and women aged 25 to 74 years without CHD at baseline, followed up for a mean 15 years after the baseline interview.

Main Outcome Measures: Measures of incident CHD were obtained from hospital records and death certificates. During the follow-up period, 1,141 cases of incident CHD occurred.

Results: At the baseline interview (1971-1975), participants completed the General Well-being Schedule from which we derived a measure of emotional vitality. Compared with individuals with low levels, those reporting high levels of emotional vitality had multivariate-adjusted relative risks of 0.81 (95% confidence interval, 0.69-0.94) for CHD. A dose-response relationship was evident (P < .001). Significant associations were also found for each individual emotional vitality component with CHD, but findings with the overall emotional vitality measure were more reliable. Further analyses suggested that one way in which emotional vitality may influence coronary health is via health behaviors. However, the effect remained significant after controlling for health behaviors and other potential confounders, including depressive symptoms or other psychological problems.

Conclusion: Emotional vitality may protect against risk of CHD in men and women.

Personality as Risk and Resilience in Physical Health

1. Timothy W. Smith

Journal: Current Directions in Psychological Science October 2006 15: 227-231, doi: 10.1111/j.1467-8721.2006.00441.x vol. 15 no. 5 227-231
1. *University of Utah*
1. Timothy W. Smith, Department of Psychology, University of Utah, 390 South 1530 East (room 502), Salt Lake City, UT 84112; Email: tim.smith@psych.utah.edu

Abstract

Research on the association between personality characteristics and subsequent physical health has produced several consistent findings and identified other tentative relationships. Chronic anger/hostility and neuroticism/negative affectivity are the best-established personality risk factors for poor health. Optimism, social dominance, and other traits also appear to influence risk. Several mechanisms have been identified as possibly underlying these effects, but few have been evaluated definitively. Future research may be well served by incorporation of concepts and methods from current personality research.

Hypertension in Older Adults and the Role of Positive Emotions

PSYCHOSOMATIC MEDICINE 68:727-733 (2006)
© 2006 American Psychosomatic Society

Glenn V. Ostir, PhD; Ivonne M. Berges, PhD; Kyriakos S. Markides, PhD and Kenneth J. Ottenbacher, PhD

From the Sealy Center on Aging (G.V.O., I.M.B., K.J.O.), the Division of Geriatrics, Department of Medicine (G.V.O., K.S.M.), the Department of Preventive Medicine and Community Health (G.V.O., K.S.M.), and the Division of Rehabilitation Sciences (K.J.O.), University of Texas Medical Branch, Galveston, TX.

Address correspondence and reprint requests to Glenn V. Ostir, PhD, UTMB, 301 University Blvd., Galveston, TX 77555-0460. Email: gostir@utmb.edu

Objective: Negative emotions have been linked to increases in blood pressure, but relations between positive emotion and blood pressure have not been investigated. Our aim was to test the hypothesis that high positive emotion would be associated with lower blood pressure in older adults.

Methods: A cross-sectional study included 2,564 Mexican Americans 65 or older, living in one of five southwestern states. Primary measures included blood pressure and positive emotion score. Data analyses included descriptive and categorical statistics and regression and cumulative logit analysis.

Results: The average age was 72.5 years, 52.8% were women, and 32.8% were on antihypertensive medication. For individuals not on antihypertensive medication, increasing positive emotion score was significantly associated with lower systolic (b = -0.35, standard error (SE) = 0.10) and diastolic (b = -0.56, SE = 0.07) blood pressure after adjusting for relevant risk factors; for those on antihypertensive medication, increasing positive emotion score was significantly associated with lower diastolic (b = -0.46, SE = 0.11) blood pressure, but not systolic blood pressure. Positive emotion was significantly associated with a four-level joint blood pressure variable. Each one-point increase in positive emotion score was associated with a 3% and 9% decreased odds of being in a higher blood pressure category for those on (odds ratio (OR) = 0.97; 95% confidence interval (CI) = 0.93-1.00) and not on (OR = 0.91; 95% CI = 0.89-0.93) antihypertensive medication, respectively.

Conclusion: Findings indicate an association between high positive emotion and lower blood pressure among older Mexican Americans. Targeting the emotional health of older adults might be considered part of non-pharmacologic hypertension treatment programs or as part of adjunctive therapy for those on antihypertensive medication.

Optimism, Distress, Health-Related Quality of Life, and Change in Cancer Antigen 125 Among Patients with Ovarian Cancer Undergoing Chemotherapy

PSYCHOSOMATIC MEDICINE 68:555-562 (2006)
© 2006 American Psychosomatic Society

Janet S. de Moor, MPH, PhD; Carl A. de Moor, PhD; Karen Basen-Engquist, MPH, PhD; Andrzej Kudelka, MD; Michael W. Bevers, MD and Lorenzo Cohen, PhD

From the Dana Farber Cancer Institute and Harvard School of Public Health, Boston, MA. (J.S.d.M.); Children's Hospital Boston and Harvard

Medical School, Boston, MA. (C.A.d.M.); The University of Texas M.D. Anderson Cancer Center, Houston, TX (L.B.-E., M.W.B., L.C.); and Regional Medical and Research Specialists, Pfizer Oncology, New Your, NY (A.K.).

Address correspondence and reprint requests to Janet S. de Moor, MPH, PhD, Dana Farber Cancer Institute, Center for Community Based Research, 44 Binney Street, Smith 342, Boston, MA 02115. Email: janey_demoor@dfci.harvard.edu

Objective: This study investigated whether situational and dispositional optimism were protective against dimensions of distress and aspects of health-related quality of life (HQoL) in patients with ovarian cancer undergoing chemotherapy. This study also evaluated whether optimism predicted a decrease in cancer antigen (CA) 125 levels during treatments.

Methods: 90 women with epithelial ovarian cancer were assessed at the start and end of chemotherapy. Optimism, distress, and HQoL were measured by self-report; CA 125 levels were gathered from patients' medical charts.

Results: Both measures of optimism were inversely associated with baseline anxiety, perceived stress, and depression. In addition, situational optimism was positively associated with baseline social and physical well-being, and dispositional optimism was positively associated with baseline social and functional well-being. However, neither measure of optimism predicted domains of distress or HQoL at the follow-up assessment after controlling for baseline levels. Dispositional optimism predicted CA 125 at the end of treatment after controlling for baseline levels. However, neither situation nor dispositional optimism predicted CA 125 falling to normal levels (≤ 35 U/mL).

Conclusion: Consistent with prior research, optimism was inversely associated with distress and positively associated with HQoL in patients with ovarian cancer undergoing chemotherapy. Higher levels of dispositional optimism at the start of chemotherapy were associated with a greater decline in patients' CA 125 during treatment.

Is the Glass Half Empty or Half Full? A Prospective Study of Optimism and Coronary Heart Disease in the Normative Aging Study

PSYCHOSOMATIC MEDICINE 63:910-916 (2001)
© 2001 American Psychosomatic Society

Laura D. Kubzansky, PhD; David Sparrow, DSc; Pantel Vokonas, MD and Ichiro Kawachi, MD

From the Department of Health and Social Behavior, Harvard School of Public Health (L.K., I.K.), and Channing Laboratory, Harvard Medical School (I.K., D.S.), Boston; Normative Aging Study, Department of Veterans Affairs Outpatient Clinic, and Department of Medicine, Boston University of Medicine (D.S., P.V.), Boston, MA.

Address reprint requests to: Dr. L. Kubzansky. Department of Health and Social Behavior, Harvard School of Public Health, 677 Huntington Ave., Boston, MA 02115. Email: Lkubzans@hsph.harvard.edu

Objective: A sense of optimism, which derives from the way individuals explain causes of daily events, has been shown to protect health, whereas pessimism has been linked to poor physical health. We examined prospectively the relationship of an optimistic or pessimistic explanatory style with coronary heart disease incidence in the Veterans Affairs Normative Aging Study, an ongoing cohort of older men.

Methods and Results: In 1986, 1,306 men completed the revised Minnesota Multiphasic Personality Inventory, from which we derived the bipolar revised Optimism-Pessimism Scale. During an average of 10 years of follow-up, 162 cases of incident coronary heart disease occurred: 71 cases of incident nonfatal myocardial infarction, 31 cases of fatal coronary heart disease, and 60 cases of angina pectoris. Compared to men with high levels of pessimism, those reporting high levels of optimism had multivariate-adjusted relative risks of .44 (95% confidence interval = 0.26-0.74) for combined nonfatal myocardial infarction and coronary heart disease death and 0.45 (95% confidence interval = 0.29-0.68) for combined angina pectoris, nonfatal myocardial infarction, and coronary heart disease death. A dose-response relation was found between levels of optimism and each outcome (P value for trend, .002 and .0004, respectively).

Conclusion: These results suggest that an optimistic explanatory style may protect against risk of coronary heart disease in older men.

Is Positive Well-Being Protective of Mobility Limitations Among Older Adults?

Journals of Gerontology B Psychol Sci Soc Sci (2008) 63 (6): 321-327.

1. Amy Love Collins
2. Noreen Goldman
3. Germán Rodriguez

+ Author Affiliations

1. *Office of Population Research, Princeton University, New Jersey*
2. Address correspondence to Amy Love Collins, PhD, c/o Noreen Goldman, Office of Population Research, Princeton, NJ 08544. Email: alc@princeton.edu

- Received June 26, 2007
- Accepted January 30, 2008

Abstract

This study examined associations among life satisfaction, perceptions of future happiness, and mobility limitations in a population-based sample of 3,363 older persons from the Survey of Health and Living Status of the Near Elderly and Elderly in Taiwan. We used zero-inflated Poisson regression to determine if current life satisfaction and perceptions of future happiness were independently related to the number of mobility limitations that developed during an approximately 8-year period. We adjusted for socio-demographic characteristics, health status, social involvement, and depressive symptoms at baseline. Life satisfaction and perceptions of future happiness were both associated with the development of fewer mobility limitations during follow-up, but only for those participants who had no mobility limitations at baseline. The results suggest a protective relationship between psychological well-being and physical decline in later life.

The Clinical Impact of Negative Psychological States: Expanding the Spectrum of Risk for Coronary Artery Disease

PSYCHOSOMATIC MEDICINE 67:S10-S14 (2005)
© 2005 American Psychosomatic Society

Laura D. Kubzansky, PhD; Karina W. Davidson, PhD and Alan Rozanski, MD

From the Department of Society, Human Development and Health, Harvard School of Public Health, Boston, MA (L.D.K.); the Division of General Medicine, Columbia College of Physicians & Surgeons, and the Cardiovascular Institute, Mount Sinai School of Medicine, New York, NY (K.W.D.); and the Division of Cardiology, St. Luke's-Roosevelt Hospital Center, and the Department of Medicine, Columbia University College of Physicians and Surgeons, New York, NY (A.R.).

Address correspondence and reprint requests to Laura D. Kubzansky, PhD, Department of Society, Human Development and Health, Harvard School of Public Health, 677 Huntington Ave., Boston, MA 02115. Email: Lkubzans@hsph.harvard.edu

Objectives: Research has demonstrated a gradient relationship between depression and the risk of adverse cardiovascular events among both initially healthy individuals and those with known cardiac disease. Moreover, recent investigators have demonstrated that adverse outcomes are even associated with the presence of relatively mild symptoms, as measured by self-report scales like the Beck Depression Inventory. The association between even mild depressive symptoms and sequelae of cardiac disease raises the following question: Is the spectrum of psychological factors associated with cardiac disease greater than previously recognized?

Methods: To address this issue, we consider a small but emerging literature that has focused on effects of other negative psychological states on cardiovascular health.

Results: Five negative states that have been linked in varying degrees to cardiovascular disease or disturbances are identified, including hopelessness, pessimism, rumination, anxiety and anger. Considering a broader spectrum of risk may help to understand more fully the mechanisms by which depression and other negative affective states influence coronary heart disease risk.

Optimism-Pessimism Assessed in the 1960s and Self-reported Health Status 30 Years Later

Doi: 10.4065/77.8.748 *Mayo Clinic Proceedings August 2002 vo. 77 no. 8 748-753*

1. Toshihiko Maruta, MD
2. Robert C. Colligan, PhD
3. Michael Malinchoe, MS
4. Kenneth P. Offord, MS

+Author Affiliations
1. *From the Department of Psychiatry and Psychology (T.M., R.C.C.) and Division of Biostatistics (M.M., K.P.O.), Mayo Clinic, Rochester, MN*
2. Address reprint requests and correspondence to Toshihiko Maruta, MD, Department of Psychiatry and Psychology, Mayo Clinic, 200 First St. SW, Rochester, MC 55905. Email: maruta.toshihiko@mayo.edu

Abstract

Objective: To study the association between explanatory style, using scores from the Optimism-Pessimism (PSM) scale of the Minnesota Multiphasic Personality Inventory (MMPI), and self-reported health status, using scores from the 36-Item Short-Form Health Survey (SF-36).

Patients and Methods: A total of 447 patients who completed the MMPI between 1962 and 1965 as self-referred general medical outpatients and also completed the SF-36 30-years later compose the current study sample. The associations between the scores on the SF-36 and the MMPI PSM scale were evaluated by analysis of variance and linear regression analysis.

Results: Of 447 patients, 101 were classified as optimistic, 272 as mixed and 74 as pessimistic. Scores on all 8-health concept domains from the SF-36 were significantly poorer in the pessimistic group than in both the optimistic and mixed group.

Conclusion: A pessimistic explanatory style, reflected by higher PSM scale scores, was significantly associated with a self-report of poorer physical and mental functioning on the SF-36 30-years later.

Don't worry, be happy: positive affect and reduced 10-year incident coronary heart disease: The Canadian Nova Scotia Health Survey

European Heart Journal (2010) 31 (9): 1065-1070. doi: 10.1093/eurheartj/ehp603

1. Karina W. Davidson*
2. Elizabeth Mostofsky
3. William Whang

+Author Affiliation
1. *Department of Medicine, Center for Behavioral Cardiovascular Health, Columbia University Medical Center, 622 West 168th Street, PH9 Room 948, New York, NY 10032, USA*

2. *Corresponding author, Tel: +1-212-342-4493, Fax: +1-212-342-3431. Email: kd2124@columbia.edu*

- Received August 19, 2009.
- Revision received December 7, 2009.
- Accepted December 7, 2009.
-

Abstract

Objectives: Positive affect is believed to predict cardiovascular health independent of negative affect. We examined whether higher levels of positive affect are associated with a lower risk of coronary heart disease (CHD) in a large prospective study with 10-years of follow-up.

Methods and Results: We examined the association between positive affect and cardiovascular events in 1,739 adults (862 men and 877 women) in the 1995 Nova Scotia Health Survey. Trained nurses conducted Type A Structured Interviews, and coders rated the degree of outwardly displayed positive affect on a five-point scale. To test that positive affect predicts incident CHD when controlling for depressive symptoms and other negative affects, we used as covariates: Center for Epidemiological Studies Depressive Symptoms Scale, the Cook Medley Hostility Scale, and the Spielberger Trait Anxiety Inventory. There were 145 (8.3%) acute non-fatal or fatal ischaemic heart disease events during the 14,916 person-years of observation. In a proportional hazards model controlling for age, sex and cardiovascular risk factors, positive affect predicted CHD (adjusted HR, 0.78; 95% CI 0.63-0.96 per point; P = 0.02), the covariate depressive symptoms continued to predict CHD as had been published previously in the same patients (HR, 1.04; 95% CI 1.01-1.07 per point; P >0.05).

Conclusion: In this large, population-based study, increased positive affect was protective against 10-year incident CHD, suggesting that preventive strategies may be enhanced not only by reducing depressive symptoms but also by increasing positive affect.

Pessimistic, Anxious and Depressive Personality Traits Predict All-Cause Mortality: The Mayo Clinic Cohort Study of Personality and Aging

PSYCHOSOMATIC MEDICINE 71:491-500 (2009)
© 2009 American Psychosomatic Society

Brandon R. Grossardt, MS; James H. Bower, MD, MSc; Yonas E. Geda, MD, MSc; Robert C. Colligan, PhD and Walter A. Rocca, MD, MPH

From the Division of Biomedical Statistics and Informatics (B.R.G.), Department of Health Sciences Research; Department of Neurology (J.H.B., W.A.R.); Department of Psychiatry and Psychology (Y.E.G., R.C.C.); and Division of Epidemiology (Y.E.G., W.A.R.), Department of Health Sciences Research, College of Medicine, Mayo Clinic, Rochester, MN.

Address correspondence and reprint to Dr. Rocca, Division of Epidemiology, Department of Health Sciences Research, Mayo Clinic, 200 First St. SW, Rochester, MN 55905. Email: rocca@mayo.edu

Objective: To study the association between several personality traits and all-cause mortality.

Methods: We established a historical cohort of 7,216 subjects who completed the Minnesota Multiphasic Personality Inventory (MMPI) for research at the Mayo Clinic from 1962 to 1965, and who resided within a 120-mile radius centered in Rochester, MN. A total of 7,080 subjects (98.1%) were followed over four decades either actively (via a direct or proxy telephone interview) or passively (via review of medical records or by obtaining their death certificates). We examined the association of pessimistic, anxious and depressive personality traits (as measured using MMPI scales) with all-cause mortality.

Results: A total of 4,634 subjects (65.5%) died during follow-up. Pessimistic, anxious and depressive personality traits were associated with increased all-cause mortality in both men and women. In addition, we observed a linear trend of increasing risk from the first to the fourth quartile for all three scales. Results were similar in additional analyses considering the personality scores as continuous variables combining the three personality traits into a composite neuroticism score, and in several sets of sensitivity analyses. These associations remained significant even when personality was measured early in life (ages 20-39 years).

Conclusions: Our findings suggest that personality traits related to neuroticism are associated with an increased risk of all-cause mortality even when they are measured early in life.

References:

(1) Erik J. Giltay, Marjolein H. Kamphuis, Sandra Kalmijn, Frans G. Zitman, Daan Kromhout. Dispositional Optimism and the Risk of Cardiovascular Death.
Arch Intern Med. 2006;1.66: 431-436

(2) Michael F. Scheier, Karen A. Matthews, Jane F. Owens, Richard Schulz, Michael W. Bridges, George J. Magovern, Charles S. Carver. Optimism and Re-Hospitalization After Coronary Artery Bypass Graft Surgery.
Arch Intern Med. 1999;159: 829-835

(3) Laura D. Kubzansky, David Sparrow, Pantel Vokonas, Ichiro Kawachi. Is the Glass Half Empty or Half Full? A Prospective Study of Optimism and Coronary Heart Disease in the Normative Aging Study.
Phychosomatic Medicine 63: 910-916 (2001)

(4) Hermann Nabi, Markku Koskenvuo, Archana Singh-Manous, jyrki Korkeila, Kakari Suominen, Katarina Korkeila, Jussi Vahtera, Mika Kivimäki. Low Pessimism Protects Against Stroke: The Health and Social Support (HeSSup) Prospective Cohort Study.
Psychosomatic Medicine 72: 134-140 (2010)

(5) Janet S. de Moor, Carl A. de Moor, Karen Basen-Engquist, Andrzej Kudelka, Michael W. Bevers, Lorenzo Cohen. Optimism, Distress, Health-Related Quality of Life, and Change in Cancer Antigen 125 Among Patients with Ovarian Cancer Undergoing Chemotherapy.
Psychosomatic Medicine 68: 555-562 (2006)

(6) Hilary A. Tindle, Yue-Fang Chang, Lewis H. Kuller, JoAnn E. Manson, Jennifer G. Robinson, Milagros C. Rosal, Greg J. Siegle, Karen A. Matthews. Optimism, Cynical Hostility and Incident Coronary Heart Disease and Mortality in the Women's Health Initiative.
Circulation 2009;120: 656-662

(7) Yoichi Chida, Andrew Steptoe, DPhil. Positive Psychological Well-Being and Mortality: A Quantitative Review of Prospective Observational Studies. *Psychosomatic Medicine 70: 741-756 (2008)*

(8) Karina W. Davidson, Elizabeth Mostofsky, William Whang. Don't Worry be Happy: Positive Affect and Reduced 10-year Incident Coronary Heart Disease: The Canadian Nova Scotia Health Survey. *European Heart Journal (2010) 31 (9): 1065-1070*

(9) Amy Love Collins, Noreen Goldman, Germán Rodriguez. Is Positive Well-Being Protective of Mobility Limitations Among Older Adults? *Journals of Gerontology B Phychol Sci Soc Sci (2008) 63 (6): 321-327*

(10) Glenn V. Ostir, Ivonne M. Berges, Kyriakos S. Markides, Kenneth J. Ottenbacher. Hypertension in Older Adults and the Role of Positive Emotions. *Psychosomatic Medicine 68: 727-733 (2006)*

(11) Timothy W. Smith. Personality as Risk and Resilience in Physical Health. *Current Directions in Psychological Science October 2006 15: 227-231*

(12) Laura D. Kubzansky, Karina W. Davidson, Alan Rozanski. The Clinical Impact of Negative Psychological States: Expanding the Spectrum of Risk for Coronary Artery Disease. *Psychosomatic Medicine 67:S10-S14 (2005)*

(13) Brandon R. Grossardt, James H. Bower, Yonas E. Geda, Robert C. Colligan, Walter A. Rocca. Pessimistic, Anxious and Depressive Personality Traits Predict All-Cause Mortality: The Mayo Clinic Cohort Study of Personality and Aging. *Psychosomatic Medicine 71: 491-500 (2009)*

(14) Toshihiko Maruta, Robert C. Colligan, Michael Malinchoc, Kenneth P. Offord. Optimism-Pessimism Assessed in the 1960s and Self-Reported Health Status 30-Years Later. *Mayo Clinic Proceedings August 2002 vol. 77 no. 8 748-753*

(15) Emmons RA and McCullough ME. Counting Blessings versus Burdens: An experimental investigation of gratitude and subjective well-being in daily life. *Personality and Social Psychology 2003;84: 377-389*

Acknowledgements

My eternal gratitude to his Dharmapatni, Yogacharini Smt. Meenakshi Devi Bhavanani and their son, Yogacharya Dr. Ananda Balayogi Bhavanani, who have all been a constant source of inspiration and guidance to me, and who continue to light the way for others with their selfless service to the great science of Yoga.